Hypothyroidism Clarity

How to transition your family

All the recipes are specially crafted to be easy, super delicious and they have been kid tested-mother approved. A family-friendly way to eat that your entire family will enjoy.

This book contains wonderfully crafted hypothyroidism recipes for your home and body that will help transform you and your family's life.

Hypothyroidism Clarity is designed to help give you FREEDOM and EMPOWERMENT. I'm sharing the EXACT STEPS I've used to overcome my emotional eating issues WITHOUT dieting.

Lose weight the way natural intended.

How to develop a powerful mindset so that you can end the self-sabotage so that you aren't starting a new program every 6 months.

How to eat more of the real foods you love and start losing weight.

Tables of contents

Disclaimer

Copy write

Dictation

Message from the Author

Quick tips to jump start your Journey

Cultivating a healthy mindset

Transitioning your Family

About the recipes

Social functions

Beyond the food: The Hypothyroidism Lifestyle

Introduction

Recipe list

Breakfast

Healthy snacks

Salads

Meat main dishes

Snacks

What has this book taught me?

Great Mess to hot success!

About the Author

Resources

Disclaimer

The information and recipes contained in this book are based upon the research and the personal experiences of the author. It's for entertainment purposes only. It is not meant to replace any advice from a health care professional. This book is meant to compliment. The reader is encouraged to use good judgement when apply the information contained and to seek advice from a qualified professional if, and as, needed. Every attempt has been made to provide accurate, up to date and reliable information. No warranties of any kind are expressed or implied. Readers acknowledge that the author is not engaging in the rendering of legal, financial, medical or professional advice. By reading this, the reader agrees that under no circumstance the author is not responsible for any loss, direct or indirect, which are incurred by using this information contained within this book. Including but not limited to errors, omissions or inaccuracies. This book is not intended as replacements from what your health care provider has suggested. The author is not responsible for any adverse effects or consequences resulting from the use of any of the suggestions, preparations or procedures discussed in this book. All matters pertaining to your health should be supervised by a health care professional. I am not a doctor, or a medical professional. This book is designed for as an educational and entertainment tool only. Please always check with your health practitioner before taking any vitamins, supplements, diet change, or herbs, as they may have side-effects, especially when combined with medications, alcohol, or other vitamins or supplements. Knowledge is power, educate yourself and find the answer to your health care needs. Wisdom is a wonderful thing to seek. I hope this book will teach and encourage you to take leaps in your life to educate yourself for a happier & healthier life. You have to take ownership of your health. All rights reserved. No part of this publication may be reproduced, distributed, or transmitted in any form or by any means, including photo copying, or recording, or other electronic, or mechanical methods, without the prior written permission of the author, except in the case of brief quotations, embodied in critical reviews, in certain other noncommercial uses permitted by copyright laws. Although every precaution has been taken by the author to verify the accuracy of the information contained herein, the author assumes no responsibility for any errors, or omissions. No liability is assumed for damages that may result from the information that is obtained within.

A.L. Childers

Copyrighted Material

Copyright 2016 Audrey Childers.

This book, or parts thereof, may not be reproduced in any form without the written permission from the Author. All rights reserved. This book is copyright protected. You cannot sell, distribute, use, quote or paraphrase any part or the content within this book without of the author. Legal action will be pursued if breached.

All rights reserved. In accordance with the U.S. write copyright act of 1976, the scanning, the uploading, and electronic scanning of any part of this book. Without permission of the publisher or author constitutes unlawful piracy and theft of the author's intellectual property. If you would like to use material from this book. (Other than for review purposes), prior written permission must be obtained by contacting the author @ permissions @ audreychilders@hotmail.com. Thank you for your support of the author's rights.

Thanks for reading my latest book. Please let me know if you need any support with it.

This Book is dedicated to my three beautiful, distracting daughters who have allowed me to experience the kind of love that people truly die for. Katlyn, Abbigail and Caroline.

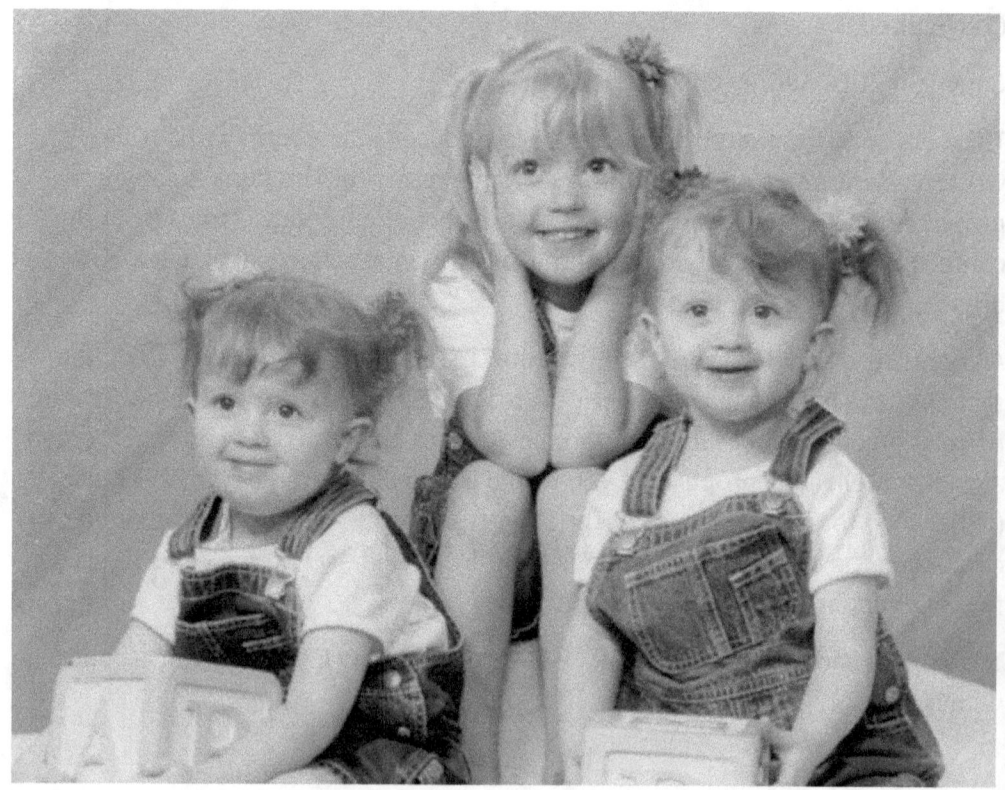

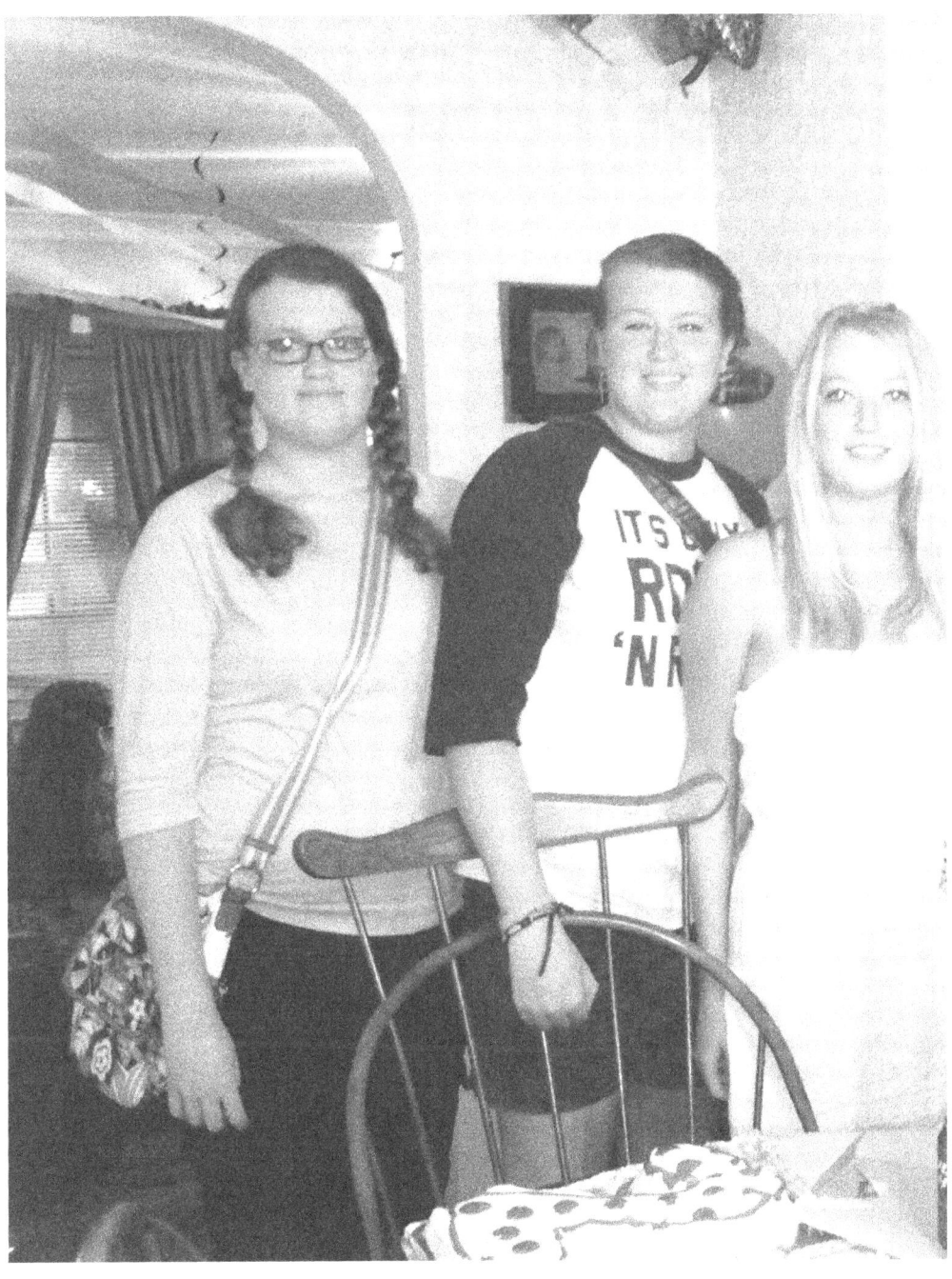

MESSAGE FROM THE AUTHOR

My goal in this book is to help you understand and show you have easy it is for you to start cutting out the foods that don't nourish your body. Hypothyroidism is a very tricky condition and complicated disorder to manage. The foods we eat can interfere with your treatment. Our body is lacking certain nutrients that heavily influence the function of our thyroid gland while certain foods can inhibit your body's ability to absorb the replacement hormones. There is no one size fits all program when you are dealing with hypothyroidism. When you start to eat smarter and are aware of what foods feed your body, despite the condition, you can start to feel better and manage your symptoms. It is my immense pleasure to write another book on hypothyroidism. In this age of overly processed, genetically modified, artificially flavored and preservative loaded foods. It's no wonder that more people are wanting to eat a more wholesome and a more all natural diet. We are trying to find our way back to the basics. I hope this book encourages you and inspires you to seek out the truth and start healing your body from the inside out. All I can give you is the blueprint of things you can start doing today to incorporate a healthier you. I am living this way. I can talk about what has worked for me and share my knowledge with you. My mission is to do everything in my power to start to heal and reach your fullest potential. To help be a source of inspiration you seek and attract what you desire with the faith that your vision of success is your destiny! You deserve to kick yourself out of that fat storage mode and into a fat burning mode. What we eat, governs what we become.

A personal favorite quote of mine is "From stressed to blessed." I mean this, believe, and receive this. I've been battling hypothyroidism for years, and I wanted to create a user-friendly handbook to help anyone affected by this disorder. I've seen many doctors over the years and none offered me ideas on diet change. I've included recipes, ideas on solutions for a healthier home, what you should be eating and shouldn't, how to shed those extra pounds, regain your self-confidence and vitality back into your life. I want you to feel strong, sexy, and beautiful. This is my heartfelt guide to you. Together, once again, you can start to gain that wonderful life that you deserve. We are all students in this thing called life. What we feel at times is not the impossible or unthinkable. Life is a wonderful journey. It's up to you to accept your journey and walk your path in life. Let's kick hypothyroidism's booty together! Thank you for allowing me into your life by sharing what I have learned over the years.

"Every time you Eat or drink, You are either Feeding disease or fighting it"

Healthy hypothyroidism meal idea's for your fast paced life.

The true appeal of eating healthy would be its simplicity and freedom. Quite often we find it hard to manage finding the time to cook a meal let alone a healthy meal. At the end of a busy day, who doesn't want a delicious home cooked meal with little to no dishes to wash? Good Nutrition is one of the best gifts that we can give ourselves and our loved ones.

This book will help you enjoy your busy life with a little more ease. All you have to do is prep a few simple healthy ingredients and toss them in a skillet, casserole dish, or a slow cooker. This is a great way for fast-paced families to enjoy a hearty, delicious and mouth-watering meals with a little less stress.

It's a proven fact that we all wished there was more time in a day. The secret to stretching your day is to make every moment count. You can do this and in the process eat amazing healthy and hearty meals from your kitchen. The blueprint breakthrough is here. All you have to do is invest in your health.

All of my hypothyroidism inspired dishes are sensational, easy to prepare and are amazingly simple. You will be able to clean up in a flash. This book will magically help you to start a new tradition.

This book contains over 100 mouthwatering recipes that can help transform your life.

You have brains in your head. You have feet in your shoes.

You can steer yourself in any direction you choose.

You're on your own. And you know what you know.

You are the guy who'll decide where to go.

—Dr. Seuss

Got Hypothyroidism? Now What.

You're crazy and it's all in your head. Which I love to hear that one- said no one ever! There is nothing scarier than not knowing why you suffer from different health related issues. What really amazes me is how easily we go to a pill to fix what ails us. You know your body, you listen to your body and you can tell when something just isn't right. There are so many potential answers as to why you can be lacking energy, can't sleep, can't lose weight, low sex drive, anxiety, aches and pains in your joints, poor hair and nail quality, premature graying or balding, constipation or hard stools, feelings of sadness, anxiety , phobia's , extremely dry skin , cracked feet and even heart palpitations. So, you've been recently diagnosed with hypothyroidism. Everyone is different. I've experienced most of these symptoms myself. You need to start doing your homework. Break out that highlighter pen and paper. You will want to start taking notes from this book and reread many time. This book will be your break through guide to getting your life back on track from book. It will help you start to breakthrough and figure out what you need to start addressing the underlying reasons to your hypothyroidism.

Remember Food is information. It's more than just calories.

You have to tailor your diet to your body's needs. Being on a very restrictive diet when you don't have to can put you at risk for adrenal fatigue and a nutrient deficiency. Nutrients give our bodies instructions about how to properly function.

First things you can do is become your own Clinical investigator.

1. Cut out gluten, dairy and soy.

People have food sensitivities and are not aware

2. Start healing your gut- start taking a probiotic, digestive enzyme and drink bone broth

Proper gut function is the key to a healthier body

3. Start addressing nutrient imbalances

Check into seeing a functional Medicine Practioner-they address the underlying causes for your disorder

4. Eliminate environmental toxins

This is household chemicals, shampoos, and tooth paste with fluoride, deodorant with aluminum, soaps and lotions these products can hijack your hormones.

5. High Stress- Your stress levels have an important impact on your hormones. You need to unwind. Stress weakens the body and makes you more vulnerable to infections.

6. Sleep- Not getting enough sleep can affect your hormones.

7. Caffeine- drinking too much caffeine will make your adrenals produce more hormones.

8. Exercise- you need to get that body moving. 30 minutes of day of anything as long as your being active. Just don't overdo it. You don't want to raise your cortisol levels.

9. Avoid plastic cups, bottles and bowls. - Bisphenol A, often known as BPA is a chemical found in hard plastics and the coatings of food and drinks cans which can behave in a similar way to estrogen and other hormones in the human body.

10. Start supporting your adrenal glands- Your adrenals produce over 50 hormones that tell almost every bodily function what they need to be doing. These hormones affect every function, organ and tissue in the body. Eating refined foods and sugars will cause a spike in your blood sugar levels, which in return cause the body to release insulin and as a result the adrenal glands will release more cortisol. When you adrenal glands are compromised this puts your body in a catabolic state. Which means your body is breaking down. Since your thyroid glands controls the metabolic activity of the body, it will attempt to slow down the catabolic state by slowing down your metabolism.

You want to start adding nutrient-dense foods that are easy to digest and have healing qualities such as

- Coconut
- Olives
- Avocado
- Cruciferous vegetables (cauliflower, broccoli, Brussels sprouts, etc.) Cooked....
- Fatty fish (e.g., wild-caught salmon)
- Chicken and turkey
- Nuts, such as walnuts and almonds
- Seeds, such as pumpkin, chia and flax
- Kelp and seaweed
- Celtic or Himalayan sea salt

11. Eat real food—not processed foods

12. Try to eat as organically as possible.

13 If you're unable to eat organically, try to eat as naturally as possible.

14. Buy organic free range eggs

15. Use organic coconut oil- Did you know that coconut oil speeds up the metabolism and supports the production of the thyroid hormone, and kills candida yeast.

16. Try to eat only fish that has been caught in the wild, not farm raised

17. Estrogen Levels – Too much estrogen slows down your thyroid gland. Try to look for a more natural form of birth control other than birth control medications. You must start ot eat organic meats. The growth hormones in meats help lead your body to unbalanced hormones.

18. Cow's milk- Cow milk is very unhealthy for us. It often contains lots of estrogen. Try using nut milk.

19. Eliminate and discard all non-stick cookware

20. Try to eat more foods with L-Tyrosine - Tyrosine is a natural amino acid which helps the body produce its own thyroid hormone. Salmon, wild rice, white beans, eggs, pumpkin seeds, chicken and turkey breast.

21. L-Arginine - Arginine is known to help stimulate the thyroid gland. It also can improve immune function, improves fertility, and alleviates erectile dysfunction. Foods that are high in L-Arginine are seaweed, sunflower seeds, pumpkin seeds, peanuts, lentils, chickpeas, chicken and turkey and seafood.

22. Avoid all sources of fluoride - As I've already stressed throughout this book, fluoride suppresses the thyroid. Drink filtered water, avoid all soft drinks, use fluoride-free toothpaste, use a shower filter, and throw away non-stick cookware. Avoid both coffee and tea which naturally has fluoride in it.

23. Eating an organic all natural diet is best - To help the body to heal itself, remove burdens on your immune system. This means that all processed foods, artificial flavors, colors, preservatives, white flour, white sugar, table salt, hydrogenated oils, aluminum and high fructose corn syrup need to be eliminated from your diet.

24. Chlorophyll - Chlorophyll provides your body with essential copper which helps to oxygenate the body, builds healthy red blood cells, and it overall assists with your skin being healthier.

25. Brazil nuts- many people with hypothyroidism are deficient in Zinc and Selenium. Studies have shown that a severe zinc or selenium deficiencies can cause decreased thyroid hormone levels. 2 Brazil nuts a day will give you your recommended dosage of selenium.

26. Coconut Oil: Buy organic, cold-pressed, coconut oil. Try to take 2 teaspoons of it each day. You can mix it in with your morning green tea or a smoothie. Coconut oil speeds up your metabolism, encourages production of the thyroid hormone, and kills candida yeast.

27. S.S.R.I. anti-depressant drugs- These drugs has fluoride as their main ingredient. S.S.R.I. drugs can be the root of nutritional deficiencies. They are toxic to your body and disrupt the serotonin that is used for digestion. Only 10% of an individual's serotonin is used by your brain, while about 80% of it is used by your digestive system. Healing your gut can solve many of your problems. Without your body being able to absorb the proper nutrients, your hypothyroidism will never be cured, because this nutrients are needed to balance the hormones and to strengthen your thyroid.

28. Sunlight- Get outside! 20 minutes of day. Let the sun hit your skin, face and forearms. Natural sunlight has many unique health benefits. 1. It allows your body to make vitamin D. Vitamin D helps regulate your immune system. 2. It cheers you up 3. Reduces heart disease 4. Sunlight kills bad bacteria. 5. Lowers blood pressure 6. Increase oxygen in the blood 7. Sunlight can help with easing the symptoms of depression.

Here are a few more quick tips to jump start your hypothyroidism health! Yes, if I repeat myself that is okay. It only means that its vital information and I want you to grasp the importance! Make sure your taking notes. Write all over this book. Highlight what you need to remember where it is easy for you to come back and access!

1. Adopt a Healthful Diet, Avoid Gluten

Your thyroid is depending on your to start feeding it and start maintaining your overall health. So stick with whole, natural, and organic foods. Steer clear of processed foods and eat gluten free. Gluten can have undesirable effects on the thyroid. If you must have bread then check out all my gluten free recipes in my book. A Survivors cookbook guide to kicking Hypothyroidisms booty.

2. Avoid Soy

Soy products have hormone disrupting effects. Soy is also high in isoflavones (or goitrogens), which can damage your thyroid gland. Products containing soy protein appear in nearly every aisle of the supermarket. That's because soy doesn't just mean tofu. Traditional soy foods also include soymilk, soynuts and edamame (green soybeans), just to name a few. Food companies also develop new food products containing soy protein from veggie burgers to fortified pastas and cereals. READ your labels. Don't worry you still can eat fried brown rice but replace it with Coconut amino's instead.

3. Iodine

Iodine is a very popular hypothyroidism natural treatment source and many natural health experts do recommend a good source of iodine. While nascent iodine is most often recommended, Lugol's brand is a fine alternative. Dr. Group's iodine supplement, is also a viable option. Vitamins C and E, D3, selenium and zinc, and omega-3s should be supplemented with your choice of iodine as well.

Some food sources of iodine include:

- Seaweed and sea vegetables
- Some yogurts (organic yogurt, Greek)
- Cranberries
- Strawberries
- Dairy products
- Dulse flakes

Keep in mind that many hypothyroidism cases are actually caused by Hashimoto's thyroiditis. It was found in some research that increasing iodine intake could actually cause your thyroid issues to worsen if you have Hashimoto's. Instead, reducing iodine intake may be the solution.

4. Eat More Antioxidant-Rich Foods

Antioxidants are also important in keeping your thyroid healthy. But rather than getting them from traditional multivitamins, that simply exit the body just as easily as they entered, obtain them from natural food sources. Load up on vitamin C from dark green vegetables and citrus fruits, Omega 3 fats from walnuts and flax seeds, and zinc from pumpkin seeds.

5. Reduce Exposure to the Chemical PFOA (Found in Non-Stick Cookware)

Finally, reduce your exposure to PFOA, found in common household products including nonstick cookware and waterproof fabrics. Researchers have found that people with higher levels of PFOA (perfluorooctanoic acid) have a higher incidence of thyroid disease. Start cooking with cast iron skillets or stainless steel cookware.

6. Coconut Oil

Raw, Virgin Coconut oil has been used as just one hypothyroidism natural treatment. Coconut oil is made up of medium chain fatty acids known as medium chain triglyceride's (MCTs), which help with metabolism and weight loss, coconut oil can also raid basal body temperatures – all good news for people suffering from low thyroid function.

7. Natural Hormone Balancing

One approach to fixing thyroid issues and hypothyroidism is the use of hormone therapy. You really need to meet with a holistic expert. There are many great holistic and naturopath doctors. Most often, synthetic hormones like Synthroid, Levoxyl, or Levothroid are used, which contain only the T4 hormone and no T3 – two hormones produced by the thyroid gland. Thyroid conditions can be serious. You should always seek a professional who knows how to help you. Our organs and glands like your thyroid, adrenals, pituitary, ovaries, testicles and pancreas regulate most of your hormone production, and if your hormones become even slightly imbalanced it can cause some serious health issues. Our gut health can also play an important role in hormone regulation. Start loading up on up on rich sources of natural omega-3s like wild fish, flaxseed, chia seeds, walnuts and grass-fed animal products. People don't boost their omega-3 foods intake to balance out the elevated omega-6s they consumed. To many mega-6 foods will cause inflammation and lead to chronic disease. Eating more coconut oil, salmon, grass fed butt like Ghee and avocados will start to provide your body with essential fats that are fundamental building blocks for hormone production. Supplements like digestive enzymes, probiotics, bone broth, kefir, fermented vegetables, and high-fiber foods can start to repair your gut lining, which also can help to balance your hormones. Caffeine will rise your cortisol levels and then it lowers your thyroid hormone levels and basically creates havoc throughout your entire body. Replace your morning coffee with herbal teas. Matcha tea is a great caffeine replacement and is loaded with antioxidants, weight loss benefits, and cancer fighting properties, heart health, brain power, skin health and a good Chlorophyll Source. Last but not least GET OUT IN THE SUN! Free vitamin D, baby. 20 minutes a day is a great way to soak up some that free essential vitamin. On the days where you can't sit out in the sun you can supplement with a good D3 vitamin.

8. Foods that you should start incorporating in your everyday eating.

Figuring out how much you need to eat for you own unique body will require time and experimentation. Eat slowly and mindfully until you are 80% full. You want to feel satisfied but not stuffed. If you exercise more, you need more calorie intake. You can easily start with a salad and add more veggies, healthy, fats and proteins to any meal. You need to make sure you're getting enough nutrients per day. Try your best to not eat 3 hours prior to bedtime and after your last meal allow a 10 hour window before you eat again. A food things you can do to start naturally balancing your hormones in your kitchen is.

9. Beneficial bacteria supports your immune system

For most people, taking a quality probiotic supplement doesn't have any side effects other than higher energy and better digestive health. As a society we have drastically cut back on our consumption of vegetables and of beneficial essential fatty acids (flax, pumpkin, black current seed oil, dark green leafy vegetables, hemp, chia seeds, fish) such as those found in certain fish (including salmon, mackerel, and herring) and flaxseed. We are consumed with little fiber and an excess of sugar, salt, and processed foods. Stress, changes in the diet, contaminated food, chlorinated water, and numerous other factors can also alter the bacterial flora in the intestinal tract. When you treat the whole person instead of just treating a disease or symptom, an imbalance in the intestinal tract stands out like an elephant in the room. So to play it safe, I recommend taking a probiotic supplement every.

Probiotics are live bacteria and yeasts that are good for your health, especially your digestive system. Probiotics are often called "good" or "helpful" bacteria because they help keep your gut healthy. Probiotics foods include yogurt, kefir, Kimchi, Sour Pickles (brined in water and sea salt instead of vinegar) Pickle juice is rich in electrolytes, and has been shown to help relieve exercise-induced muscle cramps., Kombucha, kombucha tea ,Fermented meat, fish, and eggs.

Prebiotics foods are brown rice, oatmeal, flax, chia, asparagus, Raw Jerusalem artichokes, leeks, artichokes, garlic, carrots, peas, beans, onions, chicory, jicama, tomatoes, frozen bananas, cherries, apples, pears, oranges, strawberries, cranberries, kiwi, and berries are good sources. Nuts are also a prebiotic source.

The ideal pH for the colon is very slightly acidic, in the 6.7–6.9 range. When there is an imbalance or lack of beneficial bacteria in the colon, the pH is typically more alkaline, around 7.5 or higher. The optimal pH range for gas-producing organisms is slightly alkaline at 7.2–7.3.

When someone starts taking a probiotic or a prebiotic supplement (or eats a prebiotic food), the beneficial microorganisms begin to increase in number. These good bacteria start to ferment more soluble fiber into beneficial products like butyric acid, acetic acid, lactic acid, and propionic acid. These acids provide energy, improve mineral, vitamin, and fat absorption, and help prevent inflammation and cancer. The extra acid also starts to lower the pH in the colon.

10. Goitrogenic foods which if eaten in excess can affect your thyroid in a negatively.

They are commonly known as Goitrogenic foods, which means they contain substances which can prevent your thyroid from getting its necessary amount of iodine. If eaten in excess, they interfere with the healthy function of your thyroid gland, tilting you in the direction of being even more hypothyroid, or making you susceptible to having a goiter, or enlargement of your thyroid. If you look closely at the word itself, you can see the root word is goiter (goitro-gen).

Bok choy

Broccoli

Brussels sprouts

Cabbage

Cauliflower

Garden kress

Kale

Kohlrabi

Mustard

Mustard greens

Radishes

Rutabagas

Soy

Soy milk

Soybean oil

Soy lecithin

Soy anything

Tempeh

Tofu

Turnips

Also included in the goitrogen category, even if mildly, are:

Bamboo shoots

Millet

Peaches

Peanuts

Pears

Pine nuts

Radishes

Spinach

Strawberries

Sweet potatoes

11. **Avoid Diet soda**- diet soda is a chemical cocktail made up of artificial sweeteners like aspartame, saccharin, and sucralose. Artificial sweeteners trigger insulin, which sends your body into fat storage mode and leads to weight gain.

12. **Avoid store brand Yogurt**- Conventional yogurt usually comes from milk produced by cows that are confined and unable to graze in open pasture. They're usually fed GMO grains, not grass. As the yogurt ferments, chemical defoamers are sometimes added. Then high doses of artificial sweeteners, sugar, or high fructose corn syrup are sometimes added too. That's not all: colors, preservatives, and gut-harmful carrageenan can be dumped in. If you want to eat yogurt you can make your own or call the companies and ask them what is in their products.

13. **Avoid High fructose corn syrup** - read labels, stay away from any products that contain this, it is 20x sweeter than sugar and our bodies don't recognize HFCS. What happens when our bodies doesn't recognize something? It turns it into fat. It also confuses your body & doesn't let your brain know when your full! Please, Please I beg you don't start using fake sugars like aspartame or any of those brands. They are worse than HFCS!

Have you ever stopped to think what the underlying reason why you have hypothyroidism?

Many different underlying reasons can play a role. We do know that hypothyroidism is a chronic condition of an underactive thyroid and affects millions of Americans. Environmental chemicals and toxins, pesticides, BPA, thyroid endocrine disruptors, iodine imbalance, other medications, fluoride, overuse of soy products, cigarette smoking, and gluten intolerance. All of these play a very important role in your thyroid health. A nonprofit group called Beyond Pesticides warns that some 60 percent of pesticides used today have been shown to affect the thyroid gland's production of T3 and T4 hormones. Commercially available insecticides and fungicides have also been involved. Even dental x-rays have been linked to an increased risk of thyroid disorders.

Other causes:

Iodine deficiency

Hashimoto's Thyroiditis

Certain medications eg- lithium based mood stabilizers

Viral infection

Radiation therapy to the neck area

Radioactive iodine treatment

Thyroid surgery

Pituitary gland disorder

Hypothyroidism means what exactly?

Hypothyroidism means your thyroid is not making enough thyroid hormone. Your thyroid is a butterfly-shaped gland in the front of your throat. It makes the hormones that control the way your body uses energy. Basically, our thyroid hormone tells all the cells in our bodies how busy they should be. Our bodies will go into overdrive with too much thyroid hormone (hyperthyroidism) and our bodies slow down with too little thyroid hormone (hypothyroidism). **The most common causes of hypothyroidism worldwide is dietary and environmental.** The most common cause of hypothyroidism is dietary and environmental! What does that mean exactly? That means you need to be eat to cater to your thyroid and stop using all these harmful chemicals to clean your home with and put on your body! It's not hard. Yes, a little adjustment will be needed but isn't everything we do in life for the better of our health worth a little inconvenience until it becomes a habit?

Here are a list of symptoms that Hypothyroidism can cause:

Dry skin and brittle nails

Your fingertips becoming numb

Feeling fatigued, weak, or depressed

Constipation

Memory problems or having trouble thinking clearly

Heavy or irregular menstrual periods

Joint or muscle pain

Dry skin

Hair loss

Headaches

Unexplained weight gain

Thinning hair

Clammy palms

Difficulty swallowing

Sensation of lump in throat

Dry, itchy scalp

Diminished sex drive

Persistent cold sores, boils, or breakouts

Elevated levels of LDL (the "bad" cholesterol)

Heightened risk of heart disease

Heart Palpitations

Inability to lose weight

Inability to eat in the mornings

Tightness in throat; sore throat; horse sounding voice

If you always do what you always did, you will always get what you always got.

— Albert Einstein

Author Note:

Let's not forget that we are all different. Each one of us are unique and we are biochemically individually wired and what works for one person may not work for another. We are extremely complex and each person should be valued independently. My reason for having hypothyroidism might not be your reason. Hypothyroidism isn't a 1 size fits all solution. I want to try to help you understand the many debilitating aspects of this medical condition. This book is packed full of repetitive information and is meant to be an eye opener for everyone who wants to make a difference in their lives and what some doctors just won't tell you. I want this book to be just one of your resources that is empowering to try to help you make sense of it all. We need our medical doctors, health practitioners and those who have studied years but I urge you to also find another doctor if your doctor won't listen to you or even allow you to see your lab results or even if you doctor refuses to perform necessary needed lab work.

You must realize that the thyroid has a relationship with all the hormones. It's a very complex balance and there is no straight forward treatment of just treating your thyroid alone. 1st you must make sure your adrenal glands are in total support. Adrenal fatigue is a very common amongst people with hypothyroidism. Next you have to get your cortisol levels stabilized. Having hypothyroidism your cortisol levels are already above average. Next finding the right medication for you. Everyone is different it isn't an easy one size fits all task.

Do you have weight loss tunnel vision syndrome?

How to look at your weight loss vision.

When you picked up this book, I bet losing weight wasn't your main goal. Of course, we all have that picture perfect imagine that we want to see when we look in the mirror. For some strange reason we think that our lives would be so much easier, if we could just be "that" size. If we could wear those shorts or that cute little strapless top without feeling like an escaped circus freak act. Losing weight could also mean extending your life, getting off certain medications, seeing your grandkids grown up. Whatever your **REAL** reasons are for losing weight it is an added benefit but being the healthiest you is the ultimate goal. Some of us get weight loss tunnel vision. We are so focused on the scale and our weekly weight loss "drama" that it will make you miserable and start to stress you more out where you become your own worst enemy. Emotional eating, here I come! This isn't about you losing weight. It is about you reaching your goals. Stop allowing yourself to fall back in your old ways. This is a journey. Don't focus on the scale. Focus on your weight loss vision. Focus on your health.

Why adopt a hypothyroidism diet?

Many people underestimate the importance in which their diet can have a direct effect on their thyroid levels. Eating certain foods can affect how well your body is able to absorb vital nutrients. A hypothyroidism diet is unlikely to "cure" hypothyroidism but it will certainly help to will reduce your symptoms. Eating certain foods and/or certain drinks (e.g. coffee) along with your medication can interfere with how your body reacts to the absorption and subsequently can change your thyroid levels. Most people with hypothyroidism are nutrient deficient, chemically toxic, and have a cortisol overload. Eating more nutrient-dense foods, reducing sugar intake, avoiding soy, making your own cleaning chemicals and avoiding preservatives may prove beneficial for overall health. Feeding your body with nutrient dense foods provides significant benefit in thyroid function and your hormonal biomarkers. Hormones are these little chemical messengers that are produced in one part of the body and released into the blood to trigger or regulate particular functions in other parts of your body. Your endocrine system is the supervisor. It's in charge of these network of glands throughout the body that regulate certain body functions, including body temperature, metabolism, growth, and sexual development. Understand that there are things that individually help to halter your thyroid ability to absorb your medication and you need specific foods to improve thyroid function. Our thyroid plays a most important role in metabolism. Along with your insulin and cortisol levels, thyroid hormones are an accelerating force behind metabolic rate and weight management. Many health problems start to appear if our thyroid stops working properly. Diet alone won't cure your hypothyroidism. Improving your dietary consumption by eating food that feed and heal your thyroid may also enhance T4 and T3 levels.

Why should I care about eating to cater to my thyroid or just eating healthy at all? Why all have to die someday.

Sometimes I want to shake people and say "Wake up!" You have to power to make a difference. You've always had the power. No one can force you to eat processed foods. Eating healthy isn't easy. Adjusting your life and catering to your specific health needs will benefit you in the long run. This is one of the smartest decisions that you can make. Not only will you start to look and feel better but think of the medical costs that you could be saving your future self. Not having the right nourishment makes your body sluggish, exhausted, and week. No one but you can do this. You have to be your own health advocate. Do you ever wonder what are the reasons why people are getting sick are? What is the real reason? Could it be pollution? Could it be radiation from cellular devices? Could it be global warming? Could it be lack of nutrients in our farming soil or pesticides in our food? Could it be the sneaky hidden sugars in our foods along with the saturated fat, extra sodium and tons of empty calories we consume mindlessly? No wonder our bodies are sick. The nutrients in food allow the cells in our bodies to perform their necessary functions. In other words, nutrients give our bodies instructions about how to function.

Here is a list of the top 4 causes of death in the United States. This is a statistic report from 2007 taken from the National Vital Statistics Report. None of these things may affect you directly but I am sure you know someone who it has. These numbers should scare you. You could be next.

There were total of 2,423,712 reported deaths in the United States in 2007.

1. Diseases of heart (heart disease)- 616,067 – 25.4 % of total deaths in 2007

2. Malignant neoplasms (cancer) – 562,875 – 23.2 % of total deaths in 2007

3. Cerebrovascular diseases (stroke) – 135,952

4. Chronic lower respiratory diseases – 127,924

EVERY CELL IN YOUR BODY CAN BE IMPACTED BY THYROID MALFUNCTION

Is eating to cater to your thyroid safe for your children?

Yes, real food is for everyone – children, teens and reluctant spouses. Helping your family switch from a modern American diet to nutritious, whole foods is one of the greatest gifts you can give them.

Fluoride blocks iodine receptors

Did you know that fluoride was Once Prescribed as an Anti-Thyroid Drug? Up through the 1950s, doctors in Europe and South America prescribed fluoride to reduce thyroid function in patients with over-active thyroids (hyperthyroidism). (Merck Index 1968). If you haven't already, you should invest in a water filtration system to rid your tap water of fluoride. Do we really know how safe tap water is? Look at the recent events in Flint Michigan! Can you really trust the water companies? Although fluoride concentrations in tap water are relatively low and are considered "safe" for human consumption, it is not. Fluoride has long-term neurological and hormonal affects. Fluoride is not an essential nutrient. It is also that chemical that is commonly found in most toothpaste brands. There is clear evidence that, when ingested at high doses, fluoride causes neurotoxicity. Fluoride also is understood to interfere with the absorption of iodine, possibly leading to an iodine deficiency and ultimately hypothyroidism. To benefit your health, use fluoride free tooth or make your own tooth paste. Get a good water filtration system and purchase a filter for your shower head. We use a British Berkefeld.

Natural Tooth Paste Recipe

Natural Peppermint Toothpaste

1/2 cup coconut oil

3 Tablespoons of baking soda

15 drops of peppermint food grade essential oil

Melt to soften the coconut oil. Mix in other ingredients and stir well. Place your mixture into small glass jar. Allow it to cool completely. When ready to use just dip toothbrush in and scrape small amount onto bristles.

Homemade Coconut Oil Toothpaste Recipe

6 tbsp. coconut oil

6 tbsp. baking soda

15-20 drops of a food grade essential oil (peppermint, cinnamon, grapefruit or lemon taste great)

Melt to soften the coconut oil. Mix in other ingredients and stir well. Place your mixture into small glass jar. Allow it to cool completely. When ready to use just dip toothbrush in and scrape small amount onto bristles.

Why is gluten unhealthy?

Gluten is a component of all barley, wheat, and rye products. Eating gluten can increase in inflammation, which in turn disrupts function of the hypothalamic pituitary thyroid axis (HPTA). Disruption of the hypothalamic pituitary thyroid axis decreases conversion of T4 to T3, in return changing the absorption of thyroid hormones. People have found that their thyroid function improves upon the removal of gluten from their diets.

The truth about the good fats

Healthy fats: If your diet is lacking in healthy fats, you may want to consider increasing your consumption. One of the best ways to ensure that you're getting enough fat in your diet is to eat more avocados. Avocados contain mostly monounsaturated fat and some polyunsaturated fat.

Avocados

Coconut oil

Dark chocolate

Eggs

Grass-fed butter

Nuts & Seeds

Eating more saturated fats also provides more benefits to those of us with hypothyroidism. Particularly, addition of unrefined, virgin coconut oil to the diet of individuals with hypothyroidism may: decrease brain fog, enhance cognitive performance, and boost overall physical energy. Coconut oil contains MCTs such as caprylic acid that modulate: blood sugar and metabolism, improve digestion, and reduce inflammatory responses.

Why should I oil pull?

Coconut Oil pulling can really transform your health. Your mouth is the home to millions of bacteria, fungi, viruses and other toxins, the oil acts like a cleanser, pulling out the nasties before they get a chance to spread throughout the body.

This frees up the immune system, reduces stress, curtails internal inflammation and aids well-being.

An ancient Ayurveda ritual dating back over 3,000 years, oil pulling involves placing a tablespoon of extra virgin organic cold pressed oil (I use coconut oil) into your mouth and then swishing it around for up to 20 minutes, minimum 5 minutes (pulling it between your teeth), before spitting it out. Whatever you do, do not swallow the oil as you will ingest the toxins you are trying to wipe out. Afterwards requires brushing your teeth with an all-natural fluoride-free toothpaste, and rinsing your mouth out. And you're done! It really is that easy.

Because coconut oil has been shown to:

- Balance Hormones
- Kill Candida
- Improve Digestion
- Moisturize Skin
- Reduce Cellulite
- Decrease Wrinkles and Age Spots
- Balance Blood Sugar and Improve Energy
- Improve Alzheimer's
- Increase HDL and Lower LDL Cholesterol
- Burn Fat

Your morning coffee, Hypothyroidism and your Health

Nothing like that waking up to the smell of coffee. Its gets the juices flowing with that very 1st sip. Its offer you an energetic boost and mental clarity on a feeling that life can go on.

The thyroid gland is such a very important part of the body's regulatory mechanisms; thyroid problems can affect everything in the body from our temperature to appetite to the pulse. Caffeine, a stimulant found in coffee, can affect the thyroid in a number of ways and has an effect on your central nervous system, your digestive tract, and your metabolism.

According to the recent article, in new study from the journal Thyroid people who consume coffee at the time of taking their thyroid medication, we see a 25-57% drop in T4, one of the thyroid hormones, compared to non-coffee drinkers. This adverse effect persists for up to one hour. The caffeine content within coffee inhibits absorption of thyroid replacement hormone, possibly causing you to remain stuck in a hypothyroid state even when you've been taking your medication.

Researchers have also found that for patients taking levothyroxine tablets, absorption is affected by drinking coffee and espresso within an hour of taking the thyroid drugs.

According to "Coffee and Health," by Gerard Debry, in experiments on rats, very high doses of caffeine caused the thyroid gland to enlarge, but at doses of about 300 mg, caffeine in humans did not change levels of thyroid hormones.

What about the benefits? Yes, there are many reliable studies that say coffee is full of antioxidants and polyphenols. However, these same antioxidants and polyphenols can also be found abundantly in many fruits and vegetables.

There are many other reliable studies that show coffee can play a role in the prevention of cancer, diabetes, depression, cirrhosis of the liver, gallstones, etc.

Many coffee drinkers report feeling good for the first two hours (mainly due to a dopamine spike).

(If you just can't give up that morning cup of Joe recommendations by researchers are clear: wait at least sixty minutes after taking levothyroxine before drinking coffee.) Try cutting back on coffee (and caffeine sources) for a while to give your thyroid as chance to improve. If you quit altogether, be wary of caffeine withdrawal symptoms.

Here are a few other reasons why you should give that morning cup of coffee another look: Increases blood sugar levels, Creates sugar and carbohydrate cravings, Contributes to acid reflux and damages gut lining, Worsens PMS and lumpy breasts, Impacts the conversion of T4 to T3 thyroid hormones, Is highly inflammatory and can cause insomnia and poor sleep.

What about decaf you ask?

Many manufacturers use a chemical process to remove caffeine from the coffee beans. The result is less caffeine, but more chemicals. It is the caffeine in the coffee that has the health benefits. Without it, you are left with little benefit. Coffee stimulates the adrenals to release more cortisol, our stress hormone; this is partly why we experience a wonderful but temporary and unsustainable burst of energy.

What many of us don't realize is that our tired adrenals are often the cause of unexplained weight gain, sleeping problems, feeling emotionally fragile, depression and fatigue. Drinking coffee while experiencing adrenal fatigue is only adding fuel to the fire.

Did you know that products we use every day may contain toxic chemicals and has been linked to women's health issues? They are hidden endocrine disruptors and are very tricky chemicals that play havoc on our bodies. "We are all routinely exposed to endocrine disruptors, and this has the potential to significantly harm the health of our youth," said Renee Sharp, EWG's director of research. "It's important to do what we can to avoid them, but at the same time we can't shop our way out of the problem. We need to have a real chemical policy reform."

These chemicals will increase production of certain hormones; decreasing production of others; imitating hormones; turning one hormone into another; interfering with hormone signaling; telling cells to die prematurely; competing with essential nutrients; binding to essential hormones; accumulating in organs that produce hormones. You can start avoiding these chemicals by making your own all natural cleaning supplies and being aware of the chemicals that you may purchase for your home, body and yard.

Homemade Deodorant

1/2 cup baking soda

1/2 cup arrowroot powder or 1/2 cup of cornstarch

5 tablespoon unrefined virgin coconut oil

10 drops of grapefruit essential oil or lavender essential oil

(You can pick your favorite scent. I like lavender or grapefruit.)

Mix baking soda and arrowroot together. Melt your coconut oil in the microwave in a microwave-safe bowl. Mix all ingredients (the baking soda and arrowroot powder) with the oil. Pour into clean small Mason jar. Add your essential oil to the Mason jar; close with the lid. Give it a good shake to combine the essential oil with the other mixture. By doing it this way, you can still use that bowl to eat with. Once you mix that essential oil in the bowl, it can only be used for the purpose of making your deodorant. Everything you've used is edible except the essential oils.

Unhealthy Mindset: 3 Ways we keep Ourselves Sick

EVERY CELL IN YOUR BODY CAN BE IMPACTED BY THYROID MALFUNCTION

You know that healthy habits make sense, but did you ever stop to think why you practice them?

I've heard women, in particular, say this a lot lately. They say, "Why can't I look like that?!" I will never look like that!"

Why do we mentally sabotage ourselves? Let's get something clear. You are unique. You are not meant to be me & I am not meant to be you. We are on this planet as individuals, each of us has a unique finger print that can't and won't ever be duplicated with any other human being. Ever! So why do you mentally sabotage your mindset with self-doubt and in return it starts a domino effect on your health? You are telling your subconscious without even realizing it that you are not made for greater things. You are telling your subconscious that you cannot be sexy, be brilliant and be fantastic. Be happy in your skin.

Everywhere you look — on every billboard, on every social media channel — it seems that there are beautiful, scantily clad women. So it is pushed down our throats that beauty starts from the outside but actually its starts on the inside and radiates outward.

Here's the thing: if you treat your body like it's your worst enemy – or not take ownership of your physical wellbeing – you are repelling good health. You're keeping yourself from being the best you can be in your life, because you dislike your body so much.

You're basically saying, "I dislike good health. I want to be rid of it."

Well, wish granted!

Good nutrition is an important part of leading a healthy lifestyle

You're meant to make a difference in this world; that's why you're here. But you must believe you're meant for greater things, so you can actually enter a place of mental stability, and eventually, a place of fantastic health. Don't take yourself out of the game by ignoring your bad relationship with your health.

Here are three common ways that we keep Ourselves Sick. Luckily, you can fix them.

1. **Improve your relationship with your health**

When you decide to improve your relationship with your health, be prepared for people to question and criticize you. Change can be a very difficult thing for many of us to handle. You have the mindset, to step out on faith to get the perfect health that you really wish to have. It could be from grabbing that apple instead of those chips, walking 10 minutes per day, or reading a self-help book.

Take Action: Let yourself out of that unhealthy, fast-food, over processed and artificially filled food habit because it's ruining your life.   The only way to create a different outcome is to allow yourself to forgive what's happened in the past. The past does not have to be your future. You are 100% capable of changing your future health story, so do it.

2. **You never step outside your box.**

"I can't afford eat better."

"I don't want to spend the money on a new diet book."

"I wish, someone would just give me the magic pill for my ideal body!"

"I don't want to purchase another program that isn't going to work."

Does any of this sound familiar? The more you focus on what you don't have, the less likely it is that you'll ever have it.

Take Action: Focus on what you do haveright now. Express gratitude for literally being alive. Now, you have to create a strategy to have what you really want. Set a goal, writing down realistic goals and make yourself a deadline. Take steps to get there. (And don't quit if it doesn't work the very first try.)

Or... you can keep focusing on what you lack. Call me in a year and tell me how that's working out for you.

3. **You think health is something you're granted with, rather than invest.**

You want your health to work for you, so you have to think of everything you eat as an investment. Will eating that cheeseburger build or create that healthy body? Probably not.

Will investing in self-improvement books or a mentorship program? Perhaps, if you do the work and commit to changing old habits.

Take Action: When you're about to improve your health, think carefully about why you're about to modify your life. If that item, service or experience is worth it. Then ask yourself:

Will it feel like a good investment in 90 days, 6 months, or even a year?

Will it help you create a healthier you?

Will it help create a happier you?

Will this change bring you immense joy and memories that will last forever?

Will you grow as a result?

Cultivating a healthy mindset

You don't have to repel health. Instead, build your relationship with it.

Investing in myself by joining a group program for a healthier lifestyle is the best thing I ever did for myself. Committing to my personal growth, speaking with people who has been there and done it, and finding the support of like-minded people was crucial to my success and confidence. I've created a group on Facebook called **Got Hypothyroidism**? Where you have a "safe place" to share progress and chat with one another.

It's time for you to change your health story and start becoming a healthier you! You can change the game. You can see get a healthier you and change your unhealthy past to make a better future in your life. Make the decision that it will happen for you, and work on your healthy mindset.

Take Action: **Create a food journal**. Write down everything you eat. Think about what you eat and if it benefits your body. I'm talking old school pen and paper.

Break those chains where you can become a healthier you. Once you see what you eat, you can quicklystart to know the area's in your food journal that you need to make a change.

Yes, it can be frightening. It takes a lot of courage to face your unhealthy habits in such detail. Now you can create a health plan to cut unhealthy habits and bring in the health you desire.

Investing in your health will have a high return, personally and professionally. Don't go foolishly looking for cheap thrills and expect to be in better state of health this time next year. Believe that you're worthy of investing in yourself and believe you'll have a return.

Be strong, stay positive

Transitioning your Hypothyroidism family

Reluctant spouses, kids and teenagers

An easy way to get your kids excited about their new food journey is to involve them in the process. Encourage them to help you in the kitchen – younger children can do basic tasks like washing the vegetables; older kids can help chop, peel, and clean up. Teenagers can even be in charge of the family's dinner for one night. This is a great way to teach them how to start cooking real food. Also ask your kids what they would like to eat and have them help plan the weekly meals. You can even involve them in your grocery store trip where they can add their input and help you pick out the ingredients.

You want to provide your family with all the micronutrients they need to support a healthy growing body. Raising a healthy family has its own challenges, but it's not impossible, and the healthy eating habits your children learn will help guide them for the rest of their lives. Start off slowly with introducing a recipe or a hypothyroidism friendly snack. Slow and steady wins the race.

Tips to Make Your Family Dinner less Stressful

Tips to make dinner stress free

Most of us has hit our peak time of exhaustion by late afternoon. It's a roller coaster ride of craziness. You have so much to do in the a little bit of time. After work you have game practices, errands to run, car pools, extra-curricular activities and not to mention helping your child with homework. Cooking dinner seems like another daunting task added to your already busy life.

  Recent research at Columbia University found that children who regularly had dinner with their families are less likely to abuse drugs or alcohol, and more likely to do better in school. In fact, studies show the best-adjusted children are those who eat with an adult at least five times a week, says Ann Von Berber, PhD, chair of the department of nutrition sciences at Texas Christian University in Fort Worth.

Organize in the a.m.

 Try to wash and chop your vegetables ahead of time and store them in a Ziploc® brand Bag with a dry paper towel to absorb the moisture.

Assign dinner Duties

Make an after school chore chart where your kids know and can go straight to their after school tasks. Let them know that they are appreciated and the home couldn't manage without them doing their 'special" chore. It might not seem like much but setting the table is a big deal and it is certainly one less step to take.

Onions and garlic, oh my!

Onion or garlic sautéed with olive oil can add a delicious boost any dish. If you have a recipe that needs chopped garlic or onion try to pre chop or precook it. Place them in the freezer in a Ziploc® brand Freezer Bag for safe keeping until you need it.

Snack Time

Always try to give your kids a small healthy snack while you are cooking dinner. This will help to avoid you kids getting to fussy and irritated due to being hungry before dinner.

Hanging Out

It's always fun to hang out with your family and ask them how their day has gone while you are preparing the meal and this will run into dinner time. This is a good way to stay connected in our fast pace world. This will make you family feel closer and happier when you share about each other's day. Family mealtimes are a way to increase the time you spend talking with each other and most importantly being heard in a fast paced world.

Turn up the Tunes

You can turn on some good music while you are preparing the meal. This will start making memories with you children and everyone can enjoy the music. This also can let them know that the day is over with and it's okay to start to unwind.

Slow Cooker Needed

Don't let you slow cooker just sit in that cabinet! Slow cookers are awesome little cooking machines. Who doesn't like coming home to a cooked hot meal? All you have to do is wash up and plate your food. If you need slow cooker recipes. My book A Survivors Guide to Kicking Hypothyroidisms Booty: The Slow Cooker Way has over 101 easy slow cooker recipes.

Make Ahead Meals

Prep all your meals the week on Sunday. Place them in the freezer or fridge. Where all you have to do is grab the pre prepped ingredients when you come home and start cooking. This can save you 30 minutes of dinner prep time. Always use your judgement and follow food safety practices.

Hypothyroidism in times of illness

What to do if your family is feeling sick?

Bone Broth. The new green Juice?

Today across America there a new hot trend of beverages filling cups. So what is this new magical elixir? It's Bone broth. Bone broth is loaded full of minerals and nutrients that improve your gut and digestive system. This magical elixir has been considered a great healer in many cups across the world. You have to drink high quality bone broth that is made from humanely-raised, grass-fed cows and pasture raised chickens can help start to repair the lining of the gut.

Here are 6 reasons why you should try drinking bone broth.

1. Heal and seal your gut. According to Jill Grunewald, a holistic nutrition coach and founder of Healthful Elements, a cup a day works miracles for leaky gut syndrome but it's also good for protecting non-leaky guts. The gelatin in the bone broth (found in the knuckles, feet, and other joints) helps seal up holes in intestines. This helps cure chronic diarrhea, constipation, and even some food intolerances.

2. Protecting your joints. Bone broth has glucosamine and chondroitin in it. Glucosamine has been taking as a supplement for years. Bone broth has a ton of other benefits that will make your joints happy health and pain free.

3. Better Skin. Bone broth has a rich source of collagen. Today in a world full of body imaging procedures you will see a many products with collagen. It's a cheaper to just drink bone broth with collagen and start make your skin, hair, and nails look radiant naturally from foods.

4. Mood enhancer. Several studies have shown the glycine in bone broth has improved sleeping and memory functions.

5. Immune Booster. Mark Sisson, author of The Primal Blueprint, actually calls bone broth a "superfood" thanks to the high concentration of minerals. He says that the bone marrow can help strengthen your immune system. (Something that won't surprise your grandma who always made you her famous chicken soup when you got sick!) A Harvard study even showed that some people with auto-immune disorders experienced a relief of symptoms when drinking bone broth, with some achieving a complete remission.

6. Healthier bones. Bone broth is loaded with phosphorus, magnesium, and calcium which is an essential building blocks for healthier bones.

Chicken and Beef Broth

Ingredients:

(You don't have to use both sets of bones you can use one or the other)

4 lbs. chicken bones (any combination of backs, necks, and feet)

2 lbs. beef bones (shin or neck)

2 small onions, peeled and quartered

4 small carrots, cut into 1-inch pieces

4 stalks celery, cut into 1-inch pieces

1/2 bunch flat-leaf parsley

1 bunch fresh thyme

12 oz. can tomatoes, drained

1 head garlic, halved crosswise

1 tsp. black peppercorns

Directions:

Combine bones in a deep 8-quart pot.

Rinse with cold water, scrubbing with your hands.

Drain and pack bones in pot.

Cover with 4 inches of cold water and cook over medium-high heat for about 45 minutes until liquid boils.

Reduce heat to medium and move pot so burner is off to one side. (This helps broth to circulate.)

Simmer until broth looks clear, about 1 hour, occasionally using a ladle to skim off surface fats and foamy impurities.

When broth looks clear, add remaining ingredients and simmer for an additional 2 hours.

Use a spider skimmer to remove and discard bits of meat.

Put a fine-mesh strainer over another large pot and pour broth through it; discard solids.

Drink immediately, or let cool before storing. Makes 2 1/2 quarts.

Slow Cooker Simple Bone Broth

Ingredients

3-4 lbs. of bones

1 gallon water

2 tablespoons apple cider vinegar

Instructions

Add everything to the crockpot. Cook on low setting in crockpot for 10 hours. Cool the broth, strain and pour broth into container. Store in refrigerator. Scoop out the congealed fat on top of the broth. Heat broth when needed (with spices, vegetables, etc.).

One cannot think well, love well, and sleep well if one has not dined well.

—Virginia Woolf 1882-1941, A Room of One's Own

About the recipes

All of these recipes are catered towards healing your thyroid. You won't find any recipes with cruciferous vegetables in this book. Although cruciferous vegetables are excellent for your health it has been proven to interfere with thyroid function when eaten raw. Please limit your cooked cruciferous vegetable intake to 2x a week until you get your thyroid working at the optimum level again. Cruciferous vegetables are rich sources of sulfur-containing compounds known as glucosinolates. Some glucosinolates found in raw cruciferous vegetables produces a compound known as goitrin, which has been found to interfere with thyroid hormone poduction. Very high intakes of raw cruciferous vegetables, such as raw cabbage and raw turnips, have been found to cause hypothyroidism. The reason for this book is give you the tools you need so you're not in the kitchen cooking 3 different meals. All the recipes are nutrient packed to supply your thyroid with the help is needs to support your thyroid plus everyone will enjoy them. Your family will think you're a master in the kitchen! People with hypothyroidism may feel that they have a limited selection of foods but you don't! Remember food is information. It's more than just calories. The type of food you eat will determine if you're to be healthy or sick. You must tailor your nutritional needs to your body. Being on a very restrictive diet when you don't to be can put you at risk for adrenal fatigue and nutrient deficiencies.

A diet for hypothyroidism should include whole foods rich in iodine:

whole baked organic potatoes with skin, cod, dried seaweed, shrimp, Himalayan crystal salt, baked turkey breast, dried prunes, navy beans, tuna, boiled eggs, lobster, cranberries, and green beans. Niacin-rich foods (required for normal manufacture of thyroid hormone) are tuna, chicken, prunes, bananas, turkey, salmon, sardines, and brown rice.

Riboflavin-rich foods:

Raw almonds, eggs, mushrooms, sesame seeds, salmon, and tuna.

Zinc: (as well as vitamins B6, C, and E, iodine) is a major component of thyroid hormone balance and is antimicrobial. Zinc-rich foods (boost thyroid function) are white cooked button mushrooms, chickpeas, kidney beans, dark chocolate (70 percent or higher), pumpkin, squash seeds, and almonds.

Selenium-rich foods: (helps to convert T-4 to T-3) are Brazil nuts and tuna.

High-polyphenols foods: (acts as an anti-fungal) are cocoa powder, dark chocolate, coffee, tea, flaxseed meal, red raspberries, blueberries, black currants.

Vitamin B6–rich foods: (required for normal manufacture of thyroid hormone) are raw unsalted sunflower seeds, quinoa, raw pumpkin seeds, sesame seeds, flaxseeds, pistachio nuts, cashews, tuna, halibut, salmon, dried prunes, bananas, avocados, dried apricots, and raisins.

Vitamin C–rich foods: (boost thyroid gland function) are bell peppers, dark leafy greens, kiwis, broccoli, berries, citrus fruits, tomatoes, peas, and papayas.

Riboflavin-rich foods: (or vitamin b2—essential for normal manufacture of thyroid hormone) are frozen peas, beets, crimini mushrooms, eggs, asparagus, almonds, and turkey.

Vitamin E–rich foods: (work with zinc and vitamin A to produce thyroid hormone) are raw almonds, shrimp, avocados, quinoa, salmon, extra-virgin olive oil, and cooked butternut squash.

See you are NOT limited to what you can eat with hypothyroidism. You have many options to what you can eat and why you need to be eating this. Here are more foods and **YES** you may read repeats from the paragraph above but I want you to see what an abundance of foods that you can eat. The only limit you have in the kitchen is your imagination. My recipes are a starting point. You can start to creating your favorite recipes and healing your thyroid as you eat! Your diet is part of the solution.

Fatty fish like wild salmon, trout, halibut, cod, albacore tuna, flounder, cod or sardines (omega-3s and selenium) only a few times per week….

No farmed fish, period!

No gluten.

Split peas, lentils, black beans, kidney beans, pinto beans, artichokes, raspberries, blackberries, chia seeds, red apples with skin, prunes, green peas, raw almonds, garbanzo beans, winter squash, spaghetti squash, summer squash, butternut squash, zucchini, popcorn (no microwave-ready, bagged popcorn), cherries, citrus fruits, kiwi, cantaloupe, papaya, mango, plums and red grapes, tomatoes, carrots, gluten-free, steel-cut oats or gluten-free rolled oats, watermelon, green tea, organic apple cider vinegar, lemon, garlic, leeks, parsley, celery, ginger root, tomatoes, cucumbers, carrots, asparagus, organic whole baked potatoes with skin, shrimp, Himalayan crystal salt, Celtic sea salt, baked turkey breast, dried prunes, navy beans, gluten free steel cut or rolled oats, cranberries and green beans, organic no hormone chicken, brown rice, raw almonds, eggs, sesame seeds,, chickpeas, kidney beans, dark chocolate 70 percent or higher, walnuts, cocoa powder, hempseeds, red raspberries, blueberries, black currants, brazil nuts, raw unsalted sunflower seeds, quinoa, raw pumpkin seeds, sesame seeds, flaxseeds, pistachio nuts, cashews, dried prunes, bananas, avocados, dried apricots, and raisins, red, green and orange bell peppers, romaine lettuce, kiwis, papayas, beets, all mushrooms, quinoa, extra-virgin olive oil and cooked butter nut squash. sea vegetables, dried seaweed, kelp, dulse, nori, arame, wakame, kombu, tomato paste, brewer's yeast, brown rice, algae, healing spices (Ceylon cinnamon, turmeric, gloves, cayenne pepper, garlic, oregano, sage, ginger .

Hypothyroidism at Social Functions

Hypothyroidism tricks and tip for attending a party or gathering

Macadamia Coconut Balls

2 cups unsweetened shredded coconut

1/3 cup macadamia nuts

1 banana

1/2 tsp vanilla extract

1 Tbsp. maple syrup

1 Tbsp. melted coconut oil

A pinch of nutmeg

In a food processor, process 1 cup of the coconut and all of the macadamia nuts. Add your coconut oil and pulse 10 seconds. In a medium-sized bowl, peel and mash your banana. Next add the vanilla extract, maple syrup, and nutmeg. Place the mixture from the food processor to the bowl and mix well. Using your hands, roll the mixture into one or two inch balls. Scoop up the remaining shredded coconut and pat onto each ball, coating it thoroughly. Keep your balls in the refrigerator in an air-tight container.

Fire Roasted Tomato Salsa with Cilantro and Lime

2 cans (14.5 oz. each) Any Organic Fire Roasted Diced Tomatoes, well drained

1 medium onion, chopped

2 cloves garlic, finely chopped

1/4 cup chopped fresh cilantro

1 tablespoon fresh lime juice

1/2 teaspoon coarse salt (kosher or sea salt)

1 to 2 fresh jalapeño seeded, finely chopped

In medium bowl, stir together all ingredients. Serve with Gluten free chips.

Zesty Pico

1 cup avocado, skin removed and cut into ½ chunks

1 1/4 cups coarsely chopped fresh tomato

3 tablespoons chopped onion

1/2 clove garlic, minced

1 tablespoon sliced jalapeño pepper, seeds removed

3 tablespoons fresh chopped cilantro

1/4 teaspoon salt

2 tablespoons fresh lime juice

Smash your avocado until it is the chunkiness that you desire. Next add the rest of the ingredients. Mix well to combine all ingredients in a bowl. You can use tortilla chips, pita chips and sliced fresh vegetables such as cucumber, carrot, bell pepper, celery and zucchini to dip.

Mediterranean Hummus

2 1/2 cups low-sodium canned garbanzos, drained

1/2 cup water

1/2 cup tahini

6 tablespoons fresh lemon juice

4 garlic cloves, or to taste

1/2 teaspoon Himalayan sea salt

2 teaspoons onion powder

Combine all ingredients in a food process or blender. Blend on high 1–2 minutes until smooth and creamy. Chill in a covered container before serving. You can use tortilla chips, pita chips and sliced fresh vegetables such as cucumber, carrot, bell pepper, celery and zucchini to dip.

Vine Ripened Bruschetta

2/3 cup canned low-sodium cannellini beans, drained and rinsed

5 tomatoes washed, rinsed and diced

2 tablespoons extra-virgin olive oil

3 tablespoons sun-dried tomatoes in oil, drained and finely chopped

3 cloves garlic, minced

2 tablespoons fresh rosemary, chopped

Mix all the ingredients in the olive oil. Let it sit for 30 minutes to blend the flavors. Serve on our bruschetta bread.

Cranberry Quinoa almond Butter Power Bars

2 Cups of cooked quinoa

2 Cups of gluten free uncooked oats

1/2 Cups of dried cranberries

1/2 Cups of smooth almond nut butter

1/2 Cups of almond milk

1/3 Cup of raw honey

1/4 Cup of ground flaxseed

1 tsp Ceylon cinnamon

Follow the directions and cook you quinoa as directed on the package. Preheat your oven to 350. Combine all the ingredients in a bowl together and stir until everything is mixed well.

Place in a 7x11 baking pan. Cook in the oven for 12-15 minutes.

Beyond the food: The Hypothyroidism Lifestyle

Stress:

Stress weakens our body causing to break down and allows you to be more susceptible to illness. You can have control over your lifestyle, thoughts, emotions, and stress. One of main things you can start to do is realize the sources of your stress. Sometimes we all feel like there's nothing we can do about the stress. The bills won't stop coming, there will never be more hours in the day, and your work and family responsibilities will always be demanding. That's just life. You do have the power and you can take the control over your stress. Keep in mind there isn't a "one size fits all" solution to managing stress and we all respond differently to it. I am here to let you know that you can take action and here are a few things you can do for stress management. There is a better and healthier way to cope. You can go for a walk, call a friend, take your pet for a walk, take a hot bubble bath with Epsom salt, plant a garden, listen to music, watch a funny movie, get lost in a good book, drink some chamomile tea. Another thing you can start to do is keep a stress journal which will help you identify the regular stressors in your life and the way you deal with them. Each time you feel stressed, keep track of it in your journal. As you keep a daily log, you will begin to see patterns and common themes. In your journal write down:

- What happened to make you stress

- How it made you feel, both physically and emotionally

- How you responded to it

- How you made yourself feel better

Stress relieving foods. Organic blueberries, 70% dark chocolate, wild salmon, avocado, pistachios, leafy greens, turkey, seeds, oatmeal and sunshine.

Stress causing foods. Sugar, gluten and processed foods.

Write yourself a gratitude list. Don't just list what you have. List why you appreciate what you have. Embellish them, bask in them, and be specific to why you appreciate it. Be grateful for small mercies. Only when you live life with eyes of gratitude that you can truly see the world for what it is. **Gratitude is an attitude that has a lot of benefits.**

Goats Milk Stress Bath Reliever

2 cups of powdered goat's milk

2 cup of Epsom salt

1 cup of sea salt

2 cup of baking soda

10 drops of lavender essential oil

Combine the dry ingredients and the lavender essential oil. Store in a closed container. When you are ready to take a bath, add 1 cup of dry ingredients. (Kids can use up to 1/2 cup of the mixture.) Bathe 3 times weekly, soaking for at least 12 minutes.

Epsom salt is rich in magnesium and sulfate in which are easily absorbed through the skin. Many of us are deficient in magnesium and we don't even know it. Magnesium is the second most abundant element in our cells, helps to regulate our bodies 325 enzymes, and plays an important role in organizing many bodily functions, like muscle control, electrical impulses, energy production, and the elimination of harmful toxins.

According to the National Academy of Sciences, American's magnesium deficiency helps to account for high rates of heart disease, stroke, osteoporosis, arthritis and joint pain, digestive maladies, stress-related illnesses, chronic fatigue and a number of other ailments.

(You want more body recipes? You can find them in my book: **A Survivors Cookbook Guide to Kicking Hypothyroidism Booty**)

Exercise:

Technology has made our lives simply easier. People are not as active because frankly they don't have to be. People use to have to walk to work and walk to the grocery store and just basically walk to get to anywhere they needed to be. Our modern age has given us cars to drive and machines to wash our clothes. We seem to enjoy entertainment in front of a TV or computer screen. The local grocery store have made it more convenient to purchase produce than to plant a garden. Not to mention how easy it is in our fast paced, stressed out world to run through a drive thru to grab dinner instead of slaving over a hot stove. We are burning off less calories and eating more high fat, less nutrient based foods. Exercise is very important part of staying healthy. It helps you lose weight, boost your confidence, release feel-good chemicals into your body called endorphins, reduces PMS symptoms, boost your sex drive, is a natural antidepressant, boost your self-confidence, it can help you sleep better, strengthens muscles and bones and lower the risk of some diseases. It doesn't matter what your current weight is. When you are being active it boosts high-density lipoprotein (HDL), or "good," cholesterol and decreases unhealthy triglycerides. Physical activity stimulates those brain chemicals that may leave you feeling happier and less stressed. In return, you will feel better about your appearance and this will boost your confidence and improve your self-esteem. Regular physical activity shouldn't just be based on losing weight or what you currently weigh. I want you to start to get active in your own way. One of the biggest reasons people stop exercising is they get bored with it, no support, or motivation. Try to switch it up, change your routine and have fun with it. You can start to do little things like park further away, take the stairs, take up dancing at your local community center, join a Zumba group, use your push mower, and find a partner to walk with or go window shopping. Try keeping you music playlist fresh and up to beat, set realistic goals, talk about your work out on your media platform, like Facebook, Instagram, and twitter or in Sunday school class. You can also add some competition and challenge a friend. The Bottom Line is If you get bored walking on the treadmill or in your exercise class, then stop doing what you don't like and find something that truly arouses you. Fall in love with the challenge of physical living, instead of chasing after the results of becoming fit. Take responsibility for your own enjoyment. Don't forget one major rule: It must involve some sort of spirited movement!

Body Care:

The Environmental Working Group evaluated over 72,000 products and ranked them in an easy-to-understand guide to make sure you have a resource to keep your family safe. Check out EWG's "Skin Deep Cosmetic Database" today @ http://www.ewg.org/skindeep/ . You have to start reading labels and avoiding conventional body care products that are high in DEA, parabens, propylene glycol and sodium lauryl sulfate these products are full of toxins. Plastic bottles should be replaced with glass and stainless steel due to the toxic effects of BPA. Also, change your cookware from Teflon pans to stainless steel, ceramic or cast iron this will start make a big difference in your thyroid health.

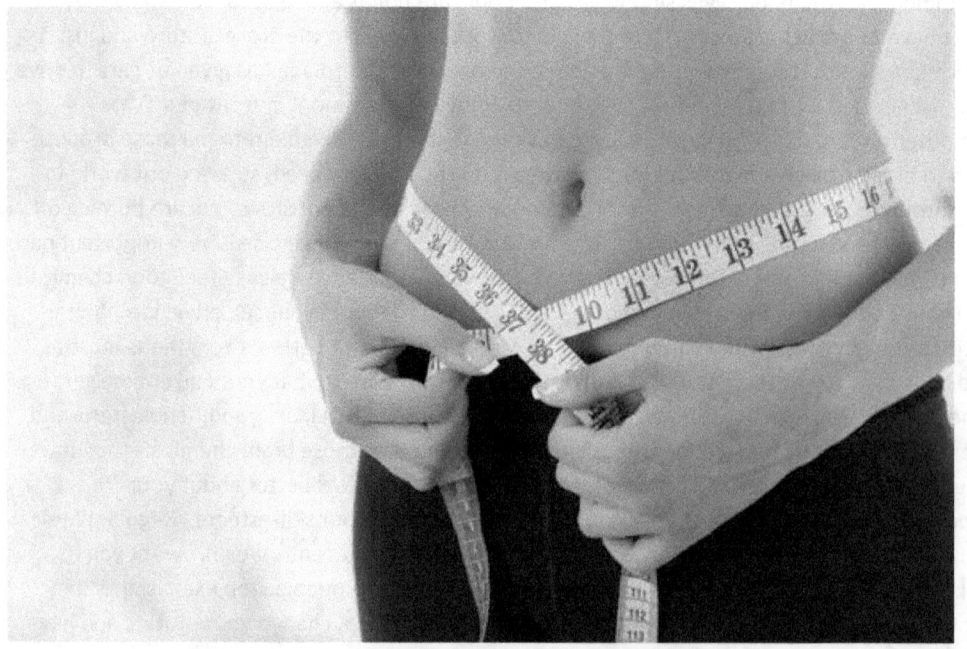

All natural hair lightener Recipe #1

½ cup raw honey

½ cup extra virgin olive oil

½ banana, smashed

Mix everything in a jar. Allow to sit for 1 hour then apply to your hair. Wrap your hair in a plastic grocery bag than wrap with a towel. This will lock in the heat. Allow the mixture to sit on your hair for 1-2 hours. The honey works as a natural high lightener. It has a peroxide affect.

All natural hair lightener recipe #2

¼ cup honey

½ cup conditioner

Mix everything in a jar. Mix everything in a jar. Allow to sit for 1 hour then apply to your hair. Wrap your hair in a plastic grocery bag than wrap with a towel. This will lock in the heat. Allow the mixture to sit on your hair for 1-2 hours. The honey works as a natural high lightener. It has a peroxide affect.

All natural hair lightener recipe #3

10 bags of chamomile tea

4 lemons

2 cups of boiling water

1 spray bottle

Boil your water in a small pot. Pour your hot water in a glass safe container. Place the tea bags in the water. Allow them to sit for 10 minutes. Take a spoon or fork and press the tea to the side of the jar to ensure you get all the chamomile tea. Next squeeze the juice of the four lemons in the container. Allow the mixture to cool enough to be safe to pour in your spray bottle. Spray the mixture on your hair as you sit out in the sun and allow your hair to dry.

All natural hair lightener recipe #4

2 tablespoons of raw honey

2 tablespoons of cinnamon

¼ cup of water

1 tablespoon of extra virgin olive oil

Mix all the ingredients and allow to sit for 1 hour. Apply to your hair. Wrap your hair in a plastic grocery bag than wrap with a towel. This will lock in the heat. Allow the mixture to sit on your hair for 1-2 hours and then rinse out. You can apply this twice a week until you get the desired results.

Can I get off my medication?

Depends on if your body starts to make T3 & T4 again. The functional optimal normal range for TSH is 0.5 to 2.5. I once was @ 175mg of levox and now I am on 35 mg's. You have to figure out what is the source that is making you hypo and fight it at the source of the issue. It could be celiac disease, Hashimoto's, leaky gut, auto immune disorder, iodine deficient, selenium or zinc deficient. A number of things can play into your having hypothyroidism. Sometimes we need to do a little bit of pruning on the branches, in order for the tree to be healthy again. So it's not just that we are, at the exclusion of all else, focusing on the root cause, but it's that we always want to do that at the very minimum. Then on top of that, we may also need to address the symptoms specifically, just for someone to feel better and function in their lives. So being on medication isn't a bad thing. You have to help your body heal itself. Keep in mind.. If TSH is above 2.5, it means your dose is too low or you're not addressing other fundamental problems, like the gut issue, the inflammation, and some of the other things that I mentioned. Recent studies have shown that the normal range for a healthy, functioning thyroid, the TSH range is 0.5 to maybe 2.2, at most 2.5, but definitely not above 4.5. If you find out that you are iodine deficient, go with foods to supplement for iodine. Seaweed, cranberries, navy beans, cod, organic potatoes to name a few...

Homemade all natural shampoo

2/3 cup of castile soap

Two teaspoons of almond or olive oil

10 drops of your favorite food grade essential oil

½ cup of coconut milk

Mix all the ingredients in a bottle. Use when needed.

Natural remedies to cure a yeast infection:

First thing is you must do is stop eating all bad carbs and sugars. Yeast feed off of bad carbs and sugars!

1. You can take an organic tampon dip it in organic yogurt no additives and insert change every 2-4 hours for 48 hours increase water intake.

2. You can take an organic tampon soak it in a diluted mixture of 20/80 Braggs apple cider vinegar with the 20 being the vinegar and 80 being purified water

3. You can freeze organic yogurt in Popsicle molds and insert in your vagina to melt while you sleep.

4. At bed time you can insert a probiotic and allow it to dissolve over night while you sleep.

5. You can douche with Kefir and add an extra probiotic for an extra punch

6. Douche with a 50/50 mixture of food grade hydrogen peroxide and purified water

7. If the lips to your vagina are itchy and irritated, apply organic coconut oil to soothe.

8. Take a baking soda bath. An entire small box of baking soda to your warm water. Sit with your legs open & rotate, move, splash the water towards your "area". Do this for about 30 minutes. Think of it as "marinating" your stuff so to speak.

9. Make sure your orally taking a probiotic

10. Start eating fermented foods

11. Drink organic cranberry juice

12. You can freeze into Popsicle molds a 50/50 mixture of organic coconut oil and yogurt. Insert at night allow it to melt while you sleep.

Eliminating Toxic House Hold Cleaners

Did you know that the products you clean your house with can cause a hormonal imbalance?

Many chemicals used in commercial cleaning products are known to have negative effects on our endocrine system. Many of these chemicals are linked to hormonal disruption and they also effect the nervous system, irritate your eyes, your skin and your airway. These harmful store bought Household cleaning products get into your system when you are using them when you breathe them in or get them on your skin where they are easily absorbed. When you use laundry detergents, fabric softeners and dryer sheets, the chemicals they contain often stay on your clothes, where they can be absorbed easily through your skin. You know that great smell after mopping the floor or cleaning that shower? Well, those chemicals leave a residue that evaporates and lingers around the home as it "off gases" throughout the day. According the Environmental Protection Agency, indoor pollution can be up to 100 times higher than outdoors, in part because of chemicals in household cleaning products. This is why you should learn to make your own cleaning products!

If you don't want to make your own cleaning products. The Environmental Working Group evaluated over 72,000 products and ranked them in an easy-to-understand guide to make sure you have a resource to keep your family safe. Check out EWG's "Skin Deep Cosmetic Database" today @ http://www.ewg.org/skindeep/

Here are few non-toxic cleaners that you can make out of your very own kitchen! If you would like more recipes please pick up my book: **The Survivors Cookbook Guide to Kicking Hypothyroidism's Booty.**

Readers are urged to all appropriate precautions before taking on any do-it-yourself task. Always follow the directions and use precautions when making your own homemade products. Never stretch your abilities too far. Each individual, fabric, or material may react differently to particular suggested use. Although this is a nontoxic and natural way to clean your home, always wear protective gloves and eyewear. Although every effort has been made to provide you with the best possible information, neither the publisher nor author are responsible for accidents, injuries, damage incurred as a result of tasks performed by readers. The author will not assume responsibility for personal or property damages from resulting in the use of formulas found in this book. This book is not a substitute for professional services.

Natural All-Purpose Floor Cleaner

2 cup distilled vinegar

2 cups water

4 cups of water

4 tablespoons of washing soda

Mix the washing soda with 4 cups of water in a bucket. Dampen you mop with the mixture. Mop well. Next, rinse mop with regular water. Pour out mixture, rinse bucket, and place regular water in the bucket and go over the mopped area. Next, place the 2 cups of vinegar and 2 cups of water mixture in a bucket and dampen the mop. Mop well.

The Tipsy Lavender-and-Lemon Bathroom Disinfecting Spray

1/2 cup white vinegar

1/2 cup vodka

10 drops lavender essential oil

10 drops lemon essential oil

1 1/2 cups water

Fill your bottle with water; add your drops of lavender and lemon essential oils. Next, add your vodka and white vinegar. Mix well. Spray on your bathroom surfaces and let sit for 10–30 minutes. Wipe off with a no microbial cloth. Don't forget to label your spray bottle with a black permanent marker.

Natural Oven Cleaner

1 ¼ cup of baking soda

¼ cup of vinegar

10 drop soft lemon food grade essential oil

2 teaspoons of liquid Castile soap

Half a cup of natural salt.

Mix the ingredients with a quarter cup of water, then put into a plastic spray bottle. Also worth trying – put a few drops of dish soap on half a lemon and use it to scrub.

Natural Furniture Polish

1 cup of Olive oil

½ of a freshly squeezed lemon

1 bowl

1 cloth

Mix both ingredients into the bowl and allow the cloth. Wipe your furniture with the cloth.

Shower Cleaner Formula

1 Teaspoon of dish soap.

1 Teaspoon of dishwasher rinse aid

1/2 a cup of food grade hydrogen peroxide.

½ cup of alcohol.

Pour each ingredient in a spray bottle. Shake well to mix. Spray on your shower and allow to sit for 10 minutes before scrubbing. Rinse and repeat if needed.

Homemade Granite Cleaner

1/4 teaspoon of liquid dish soap

1/4 cup of rubbing alcohol

2 1/2 cups of water

Pour all the ingredients in a spray bottle and shake to mix. Spray on your granite counter and make sure you rinse it well with a clean cloth with only water on it.

Carpet Stain Remover

1 cup of water

1 cup of vinegar

Mix the ingredients in a spray bottle and spray on the carpet stain. Allow to sit for a few minutes and carefully dab up.

Heavy Duty Carpet Cleaner

1/4 cup of salt

¼ cup of vinegar

1/4 cup of borax

Mix well and rub into the carpet in a circular motion. Use clean water to help wipe the mixture away.

Home Made Windex

1/4 Cup (4oz) Isopropyl Rubbing Alcohol

Pour the alcohol into a spray bottle and spray on your window. Wipe clean with a cloth.

Home-Made Febreze

¼ cup water

20 drops of your favorite essential oil

Place in a plastic spray bottle, fill the remaining space with hot water and give it a shake.

Toilet Cleaner

10 drops of Lavender Essential Oil

10 drops of Tea Tree Oi.

1/3 cup of white vinegar

1/3 cup of baking soda

Place the baking soda in the toilet, next add your drops of essential oils and finally pour in your vinegar. Allow to sit for 20 minutes next scrub the mixture and flush.

Natural Bleach Alternative

6 cups water

1/4 cup fresh lemon juice

1 cup of food grade hydrogen peroxide

Pour the mixture in a safe container to store in your laundry room. You can add ½-1 whole cup per load and this can be used as a household cleaner.

Natural Disinfectant Cleaning Wipes Alternative

1/4 cup of vinegar

1 cup of water

10 drops of eucalyptus essential oil

10 drops of lemon essential oil

7 drops of tea tree essential oil

Mix the solution in a spray bottle. Spray on the surface of what you want disinfected and wipe clean with some old cut up clothes.

You can burn White Sage Smudge Sticks. This herb that cleanses, purifies and heals the body. By burning white sage, you can expect to see and smell white smoke billowing out from it creating a festive and herbal delight. You can buy natural white sage bundles easily off of Amazon or on my blog page **Thehypothyroidismchick.com** look @ my blog post **Easy and simple Natural Ways to Make Your House Smell like Christmas.**

Stovetop Potpourri

Ingredients:

2 cups fresh cranberries

3 tangerines, halved

3 whole cinnamon sticks

2 star anise

1 teaspoon whole cloves

1 vanilla bean + 1 tablespoon vanilla extract

1 small branch fresh pine

1 cup pomegranate

Water

Combine all ingredients in pot, filling 3/4 of the pot with water. Bring to boil, then turn down heat and allow to simmer for at least 4 hours. Continue to add water to the pot, as the liquid evaporates. You can let the pot cool down overnight, and reheat and simmer the next day, for a full weekend of Christmas goodness.

Crock Pot Simmer

1 orange sliced

2 cups of water

2 tablespoon of vanilla extract

4 cinnamon sticks

Combine all ingredients in your crockpot and allow to slowly cook on low. Your house will smell amazing. You can also make this recipe on the stove.

Homemade Potpourri

Ingredients

Cloves

Cinnamon sticks

Star anise

Oranges

Apples

Pine cones

Instructions

1. Preheat oven to 250 degrees. Slice apples and oranges thin, really thin. Place in a single layer on cookie sheets and bake for an hour and a half, check every half hour thereafter. Once dry, mix with your spices. Jar and allow to "marinate" for a day. Place this in a bowl to make your house smell fantastic!

Natural Room deodorizer

1 cup of coffee grounds

Place you coffee grounds in a bowl, cup or container with a lid that has holes in the top. The coffee will absorb orders. Replace and throw away often.

Natural Room Freshener

Your favorite essential oil

(Rosemary, vanilla and lemon is a nice smelling combo)

Cotton balls

Small container

Place a cotton ball in a small container and add 15 drops of your favorite essential oil. Place this around your home. Also, every time you replace your air filter, add 10-15 drops of your favorite essential oil and this will make your entire house smell good. You can also place a few drops on a light bulb.

Homemade Air Freshener

Small Mason Jars

Cloth

Baking soda

Essential oil

Fill your mason jar half way with baking soda. Add 15 drops of your favorite essential oils. Lay the fabric across the lid of the jar and place the ring of the jar to seal it. You want the fabric just big enough to be able to seal the jar and cut a few slits in the cloth.

All natural Room Spray

This non-toxic alternative will have your home smelling great in no time!

10-20 drops of your favorite Essential oils

1 clean spray bottle 16 oz. of distilled water

Pour the water in your spray bottle and then add your essential oil.

Store in dark, cool place and shake it before use. You can spray on furniture, linens or in the air to refresh your home.

Natural Carpet Cleaner

Baking Soda

Sprinkle baking soda on any carpet and allow to sit 20 minutes. Vacuum the baking soda up and it will help release dirt and orders from your carpet.

Grease Cutting floor cleaner

1/4 cup vinegar

1 tablespoon of dawn dish soap

¼ cup washing soda

Add your ingredients to a bucket that is half way full of water. Once you blend it, it will become full of bubbles. It does go away and dry very well.

Shower and Tub Cleaner

Spray bottle

1 cup of vinegar

1 cup of dawn dish detergent

You want equal amounts of each. Pour in your spray bottle and label it. Spray on your shower or tub and allow it to sit for 1 hour then proceed to scrub the area and rinse well.

This homemade laundry detergent recipe not only keeps those harsh chemicals away, but it's also cheaper, lasts longer, and made with all-natural ingredients; it's a greener, healthier alternative to commercial chemically loaded products. There's nothing more natural or better than natural products like vinegar, baking soda, and essential oils.

Homemade Powder Laundry Soap

I mix mine in a large bucket then pour it in a large glass container with a 1/4 small scoop. Only 3 ingredients to make this detergent! Add 3 cups each of the washing soda and borax detergent booster. Mix well. Grate one bar of FELS-NAPTHA soap in a bowl. (Any castile soap or ivory soap will work too.) All you need is 1/4 of a cup for each load, and this is exactly the scoop size that I use. Makes things easier for me. Your laundry will be fresh, clean, and actually smell good.

Vinegar of the Four Thieves Insect Repellent Ingredients****

- 1 32 ounce bottle of Apple Cider Vinegar
- 2 TBSP each of dried Sage, Rosemary, Lavender, Thyme and Mint
- At least quart size glass jar with airtight lid

How to Make the Vinegar of the Four Thieves Insect Repellent

Pour your vinegar and dried herbs into large glass jar. Seal it tightly and store it in a place where you can see it daily to shake it for 2 weeks. After 2 weeks, strain the herbs out and store in spray bottles and keep in the fridge. When you use it on your skin, dilute to half with water in a spray bottle and use as needed.

All natural wasps trap

1/4 cup vinegar

1/2 cup of warm water

1/2 cup sugar

1 teaspoon salt

Mix this solution in an open container, place where needed. Make sure it is out of the hands of children. Although it's nontoxic they might still be able to get stunk if they put their hands in the container.

Fermented Foods

A healthy gut plays a significant role in hormone regulation. Having a leaky gut or a lack of probiotic foods lining your intestinal wall can help cause a hormonal imbalance. For most of us, taking a quality probiotic supplement doesn't have any side effects other than higher energy and better digestive health. As a society we have drastically cut back on our consumption of vegetables and of beneficial essential fatty acids (flax, pumpkin, black current seed oil, dark green leafy vegetables, hemp, chia seeds, fish) such as those found in certain fish (including salmon, mackerel, and herring) and flaxseed. We are consume little fiber to no fiber and eat an excess of sugar, salt, and processed foods. Stress, changes in the diet, contaminated food, chlorinated water, and numerous other factors can also alter the bacterial flora in the intestinal tract. When you treat the whole person instead of just treating a disease or symptom, an imbalance in the intestinal tract stands out like an elephant in the room. So to play it safe, I recommend taking a probiotic supplement every. Along with eating fermented foods.

Probiotics are live bacteria and yeasts that are good for your health, especially your digestive system. Probiotics are often called "good" or "helpful" bacteria because they help keep your gut healthy. Probiotics foods include yogurt, kefir, Kimchi, Sour Pickles (brined in water and sea salt instead of vinegar) Pickle juice is rich in electrolytes, and has been shown to help relieve exercise-induced muscle cramps., Kombucha, kombucha tea ,Fermented meat, fish, and eggs.

Prebiotics foods are brown rice, oatmeal, flax, chia, asparagus, Raw Jerusalem artichokes, leeks, artichokes, garlic, carrots, peas, beans, onions, chicory, jicama, tomatoes, frozen bananas, cherries, apples, pears, oranges, strawberries, cranberries, kiwi, and berries are good sources. Nuts are also a prebiotic source. All these foods that I have listed is hypothyroidism friendly.

The ideal pH for the colon is very slightly acidic, in the 6.7–6.9 range. When there is an imbalance or lack of beneficial bacteria in the colon, the pH is typically more alkaline, around 7.5 or higher. The optimal pH range for gas-producing organisms is slightly alkaline at 7.2–7.3.

When someone starts taking a probiotic or a prebiotic supplement (or eats a prebiotic food), the beneficial microorganisms begin to increase in number. These good bacteria start to ferment more soluble fiber into beneficial products like butyric acid, acetic acid, lactic acid, and propionic acid. These acids provide energy, improve mineral, vitamin, and fat absorption, and help prevent inflammation and cancer. The extra acid also starts to lower the pH in the colon.

Homemade Raw Kombucha Fermented Applesauce

Ingredients

5-6 apples

1/4 cup kombucha - can be plain or flavored.

Instructions

Peel, core, and slice apples. Place in food processor and puree. Add kombucha and puree until you reach desired consistency. Place in sealed mason jar and leave on the counter for 24 hours. Store in fridge. This will stay good for 1 month.

When you decide that this isn't about losing weight it's about being the healthiest you that you can be, then you're ready for action and you will likely succeed!

SALT

The Dietary Guidelines for Americans recommend limiting sodium to less than 2,300 mg a day—or 1,500 mg if you're age fifty-one or older or if you are black or if you have high blood pressure, diabetes, or chronic kidney disease. Read labels; it seems everything has sodium in it. Our bodies are on a sodium overload!

Pink Himalayan salt is naturally rich in iodine, so it doesn't need to be artificially added in. It also helps to create an electrolyte balance in your body, increases hydration, regulates water content both inside and outside of cells, balance pH (alkaline/acidity), and help to reduce acid reflux, prevents muscle cramping, aids in proper metabolism functioning, strengthen bones, lower blood pressure, help the intestines absorb nutrients, prevent goiters, improve circulation, dissolve and eliminate sediment to remove toxins. So, how much is 1,500 mg of salt? It is ¾ of a teaspoon.

Unbelievable!

Another thing many hypothyroid sufferers deal with is the lack of iodine in their body. Iodine is a critical essential trace element in our diet. Our bodies can't make iodine; therefore we have to rely on food to obtain it. This essential trace element is an absolute necessity for normal growth and development. In the year 1924, the Morton Salt Company, at the request of the government, historically started to add iodine to their salt mixture (in the form of potassium iodide). Table salt that you buy out of the store is bad for you anyway. "Table salt" has a list of other hidden chemicals. These chemicals include everything from manufactured forms of sodium solo-co-aluminate, iodide, sodium bicarbonate, fluoride, anticaking agents, toxic amounts of potassium iodide, and aluminum derivatives. So, the next time you go to grab that saltshaker, think of all the other little things you could be getting along with it. I'm here to shout it out to you! **You don't have to rely solely on salt to get your iodine.** But if you insist on "salting" your foods, go a must healthier, more natural route—Himalayan sea salt or Celtic sea salt. The benefits of getting enough iodine is that your metabolism will be able to function more properly. We are on a sodium overload with all the processed foods. Read labels. Watch your sodium intake from prepackaged foods. Try to avoid prepackaged foods. **Good rule of thumb: if it came from a plant, eat it; if it was made in a plant, don't.** You have plenty of food options to pick from that are naturally high in iodine. They range from seafood to potatoes, and it's nice to be able to have a variety of different foods. Even better news: everything on this list, you can eat to help your thyroid become healthier. Our bodies need an average of 150 micrograms of iodine per day.

1 medium baked organic potato with skin, 60 micrograms of iodine

Dried seaweed (1/4 ounce), 4,500 micrograms of iodine

Cod fish (3 ounces), 99 micrograms of iodine

Shrimp (3 ounces), 35 micrograms of iodine

Himalayan crystal salt (1/2 gram), 250 micrograms of iodine

Baked turkey breast (3 ounces), 34 micrograms of iodine

Dried prunes (5 prunes), 13 micrograms of iodine

Navy beans (1/2 cup), 32 micrograms of iodine

Fish sticks (2 fish sticks), 35 micrograms of iodine

Tuna in water (3 ounces), 17 micrograms of iodine

Boiled eggs (1 large egg), 12 micrograms of iodine

Plain yogurt (1 cup), 154 micrograms of iodine

Bananas (1 medium banana), 3 micrograms of iodine

Lobster (100 grams), 100 micrograms of iodine

Cheddar cheese (1 ounce), 12 micrograms of iodine

Cranberries (4 ounces), 400 micrograms of iodine

Green beans (1/2 cup), 3 micrograms of iodine

Never lose an opportunity of urging a practical beginning, however small, for it is wonderful how often in such matters the mustard-seed germinates and roots itself.

—Florence Nightingale

Breakfast

Breakfast is the most important meal of the day. Breakfast" literally means the meal that "breaks the fast". You've been sleeping all night fasting. Your body needs to be rebooted. You've got to "jump-start" that metabolism. Eating a healthy breakfast has been medically proven to have many health benefits, including weight control , reducing the risk of obesity , it certainly will boost your fiber intake to help you reach your daily goal of 20 to 35 grams (for adults). Eating breakfast has been shown to improve performance, have heart health advantages, helps you avoid fluctuating glucose levels, which can lead to diabetes later in life, helps you consume less calories throughout the day, so you're not binge eating of starvation at lunch time. It will give you that mental edge by enhancing your memory, your clarity, and the speed in which you are processing information, your reasoning skills, your creativity and how you absorb information. Scientists at the University of Milan in Italy reviewed 15 studies and found some evidence that those benefits. One theory suggested that if you eat a healthy breakfast it can reduce hunger throughout the day, and help you make better food choices at other meals. You should eat no later than 2 hours of waking up. Also, if you skip breakfast your hunger hormones are boosted and it can also throw your body into survival mode. Which in return starts breaking down protein in your muscles and your muscles will slowly start to break down.   Now, I hope you see the importance of why eating a healthy breakfast is so important.

Feed your family and get them out the door in a flash with these family-friendly breakfasts. Some of these you can make ahead and let the kids help you prepare it.

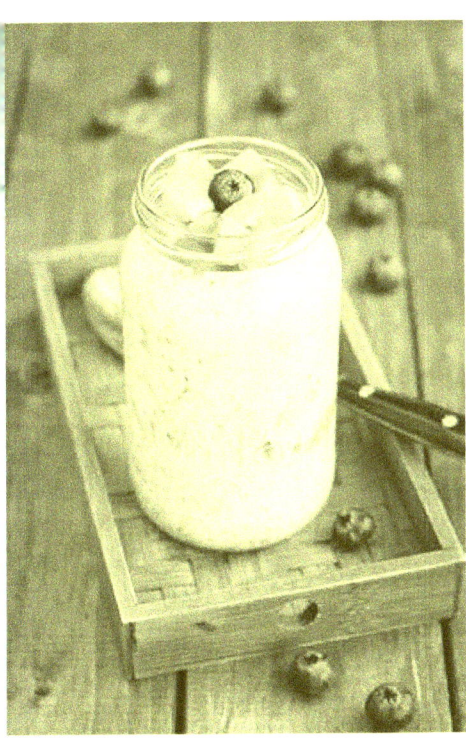

Banana Chocolate Overnight Oats

2 cups GF steel cut or rolled oats (steel cut for a crunch or rolled oats for a smoother oatmeal)

1 1/2 cups of almond or coconut milk

1/2 cups almond or coconut yogurt

1–2 tablespoon cocoa

1 tablespoon of ground flaxseed (omega-3 fatty acids)

1 tablespoon raw honey or grade B maple syrup Pour the mixture into two 8-ounce mason jars with lids, seal tightly, and refrigerate for at least 6 hours, preferably overnight. When ready to eat, give the oats a good shake and dig in!

Honey-Lime Fruit Salad

This easy-to-make breakfast is full of vitamins and antioxidants

2 cups chopped seasonal fruits

(I use red grapes, kiwis, mandarins, and bananas)

1 teaspoon lime juice

1 tablespoon organic honey

Combine all the ingredients in a mixing bowl.

Vegetable Quiche

1 bell pepper

2 red onions

1/2 zucchini

3 eggs

1 clove garlic, minced

Fresh parsley leaves (a handful)

3 tablespoon raw, unfiltered coconut oil

Preheat oven to 350°F. Chop vegetables and sauté in 1 1/2 tbsp. oil on medium heat for 3–4 minutes then add to a well-oiled oven-proof dish. Mix parsley, garlic and eggs in a bowl. Now pour over the vegetables and bake for 25 minutes or until firm in the center.

Mini Apple Crisp

1 medium organic apple

1 tablespoon brown sugar

1 tablespoon oats

1/2 teaspoon cinnamon

Heat oven to 350°F. Peel and core the apple and chop into 1/4-inch squares. Mix in a small bowl with sugar, oats, and cinnamon and put into a small baking dish, or line a muffin pan with paper cups. Bake for 15 minutes.

3-Ingredient Pancake Mix

1 banana

2 eggs

1 teaspoon of Ceylon cinnamon

2 tablespoons of Earth Balance butter

Mix all ingredients. Melt butter in a cast-iron skillet. Pour silver-dollar-size amounts of batter in pan. Cook 60 seconds and flip to cook the other side.

Morning Milkshake

What kid doesn't want to have a milk shake for breakfast? This is an easy and way to sneak a healthy meal!

1 cup almond milk

1 tablespoon raw honey

1 tablespoon all natural peanut butter or almond butter

1 banana, frozen (or fresh bananas and add a handful of ice cubes)

1/4 tsp. cinnamon

1 tablespoon of freshly ground flax seeds or prepared grounded flax seed mill

Combine all ingredients in a blender and blend until smooth.

Green "Thank the Goddess" Smoothie

1 cup cucumber chunks, peeled

1/2 avocado, peeled and cut into chunks

1 large kiwi, peeled and cut into chunks

1/2 cup fresh OJ

1/4 cup of fresh mint leaves

1 cup of romaine lettuce

4 pitted, dried apricots

5 ice cubes

This a delicious, easy drink to make. Add all ingredients into the blender and voila! If it's too thick, add some more freshly squeezed OJ.

Happy-Skin Smoothie

Try something different: freeze 1/2 cup of pure pumpkin (not pumpkin pie mix) in an ice cube tray.

1/2 cup of ice-cubed pure pumpkin

7 oz of So Delicious Greek-style coconut milk yogurt

1/2 cup of vita coconut water

2 tablespoons of flaxseed meal

1/2 teaspoon pumpkin spice pie mix

This a delicious, easy drink to make. Add all ingredients into the blender and voila! Your skin, thyroid, and body will thank you. And voila!

Cranberry Orange Steel Cut Oats

3 cups water

1 cup almond milk

1 tablespoon coconut oil

1 cup gluten free steel-cut oats

Sprinkle of Himalayan salt

Juice and zest from one whole orange

1/2 cup cranberries, crushed

Top with raw pumpkin seeds

Add your water and milk in a large saucepan. Simmer over medium heat. Next melt the coconut oil in a 12-inch skillet over medium heat. Add your oats and toast, stirring occasionally, until golden and fragrant, around 1½ to 2 minutes. Stir in your oats into the simmering water/milk mixture. Reduce your heat to medium low and simmer gently for about 20 minutes, cook until the mixture is very thick. Add the salt. Continue to cook the mixture, stirring frequently, for about 10 minutes or until almost all the liquid is absorbed. Mix in the orange juice and zest. Ladle in to bowls and top with cranberries and raw pumpkin seeds.

Almond oatmeal

½ cup no sugar applesauce

2 tablespoons almond butter

2 tablespoons coconut milk

Dash of cinnamon

Dash of nutmeg

Put all ingredients in a small saucepan over med heat. Allow it to cook until done for about 10 minutes. This would be great topped with bananas and chopped Brazil nuts.

Mushroom-stuffed Omelet

I love eating breakfast for dinner. Having mushrooms, onions, and eggs are a great way to boost selenium levels. Here is a quick recipe that is both filling and super easy to whip up.

Ingredients:

4 organic or cage free eggs

3 medium-sized mushrooms, diced

½ tablespoon coconut oil or ½ tablespoon of avocado oil

A teaspoon of dairy free and soy free butter

Salt and pepper to taste

Directions:

In a cast iron skillet add a ½ tablespoon of coconut oil or avocado oil and sauté the mushrooms till they are golden brown. While mushrooms are browning.

Whisk eggs with seasonings in a bowl. After the mushrooms have browned. Add the teaspoon of butter. Stir the butter around the pan so it can get completely coated and mixed with the mushrooms.

Add the egg mixture, it will take about 1 minute for the egg to set and then flip over. Heat for another 30 seconds, then remove from pan. Place on a plate.

Overnight Pumpkin Pie Chia Pudding

2 cups coconut milk

1 cup cooked pumpkin puree

3 TBS grade B maple syrup OR raw honey

1 tsp vanilla extract

½ tsp cinnamon powder

¼ tsp ginger powder

¼ tsp allspice

4 TBS chia seeds

OPTIONAL TOPPING

Fresh fruit

Shredded coconut

Place all ingredients, except for chia seeds, into a blender and puree until smooth. Place the chia seeds into a mason jar, pour pumpkin pie flavored liquid over seeds. Seal the Mason jar with a lid and shake it good to mix well. Place in fridge the night and the next morning you will have amazing pumpkin pie pudding.

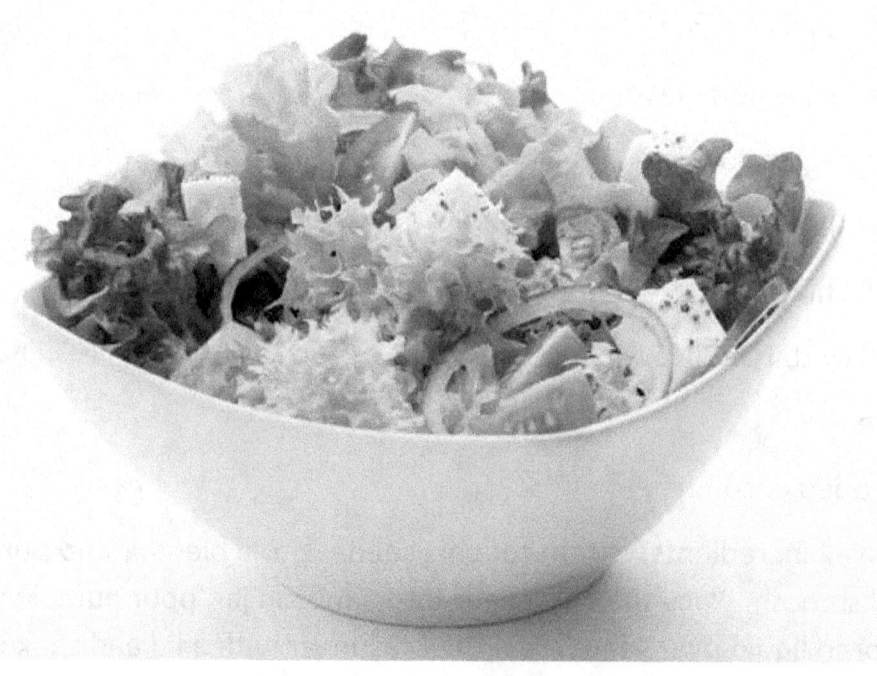

Soups and Salads

Eat salads in place of meals as much as possible. You can make your salads crispy, chewy, colorful and fun to eat. Most people enjoy eating salads--even kids! It's hard to believe that something we can't even digest can be so good for us! Eating a high-fiber diet can help lower cholesterol levels and prevent constipation. There is plenty of evidence that nutrient-rich plant foods contribute to overall health. Adding little good fat found in olive oil, avocado and nuts along with your vegetables helps your body absorb protective phytochemicals, like lycopene from tomatoes and lutein from dark green vegetables. This combination of vitamins supports the immune system, protects bones and keeps the cardiovascular system healthy.

You want to stick to homemade vinaigrettes, which are very easy to make. A great, easy-to-remember ratio is 1 part acid to 1 part oil. You don't even have to measure it if you're using a glass jar or container. Just size up an equal measure of each, then add a teaspoon or two of Dijon mustard. You can also add a dash of some salt and pepper to your taste, put on the lid, and shake. Make enough dressing to flavor your salad without drowning them in dressing. Try to experiment with different citrus juices, vinegars, flavored salts, and mustards, even a little honey. Try using your blender to make bigger batches of vinaigrette involving ingredients you'd normally have to chop like herbs, peppers, or capers. Your healthy homemade dressing will keep in the fridge for up to two weeks in a tightly sealed jar.

Chickpea Veggie Salad-in-a-Jar

This fills one 32 oz. Mason jar. Make sure to wash & dry your veggies before using.

1 oz. goat cheese

½ cup cooked, cold quinoa

1 bell pepper, chopped

1 cucumber, chopped

4 oz. grape or cherry tomatoes

5 oz. chickpeas, rinsed & dried

Dressing:

3 tsp olive oil

1 tsp white vinegar

Splash of lemon juice

Sprinkle of black pepper

Whisk dressing in a small bowl, then transfer to the bottom of the jar. Layer chickpeas on dressing. Add tomatoes, add cucumber, add bell pepper, add quinoa and top with goat cheese. Secure lid on tightly until ready to eat. Shake the salad just before eating.

Layered Quinoa Salad-in-a-Jar

This fills one 32 oz. Mason jar. Make sure to wash & dry your veggies before using.

3 Tbsp. avocado cilantro-Lime Vinaigrette

½ cup black beans, rinsed & dried

¼ cup cherry tomatoes

½ of a green pepper, chopped

½ cup cooked, cold quinoa

¼ cup organic romaine lettuce

Place the dressing in the bottom of the jar. Next add the black beans, add the tomatoes, add the peppers, add the quinoa and then add the chopped romaine. Try not to pack it in too tight, or you won't have room to shake the dressings when you are ready to eat. Seal the lid on & store in the fridge. When ready (with the lid on) shake the jar to mix everything.

Avocado Cilantro Lime Vinaigrette

½ cup extra-virgin olive oil

1 cup cilantro

¼ tsp of minced garlic

The juice of 1 orange

The juice of 3 limes

1 avocado

Salt & pepper to taste

Combine all ingredients into a blender or food processor

Puree until smooth

Mediterranean Quinoa with Seasonal Vegetables Salad-in-a-jar

This fills one 32 oz. Mason jar. You could divide this up into smaller jars. Make sure to wash & dry your veggies before using.

1 cup quinoa, rinsed well

2 cups vegetable broth

1 zucchini, diced

1 cup of corn

½ cup cherry tomatoes, diced

¼ cup red onion, diced

Vinaigrette:

2 teaspoons whole grain mustard

3 tablespoons freshly squeezed lemon juice

1 tablespoon Bragg's organic apple cider vinegar

2 garlics clove, finely minced

1/4 teaspoon crushed red pepper flakes

Freshly ground black pepper to taste

1/2 cup extra-virgin olive oil

Roast zucchini and onions, uncovered, for 20 minutes. Stir vegetables and add tomatoes and corn. Continuing roasting until tomatoes collapse, about 10 minutes. Remove vegetables and set aside

Vinaigrette

In a medium bowl whisk together mustard, lemon juice, Braggs vinegar, garlic, red pepper flakes, salt and pepper. Gradually whisk in olive oil.

Place 3 tablespoons of the dressing in the bottom of the mason jar.

Next place the roasted cooled veggies on top of the dressing and add the quinoa. Try not to pack it in too tight, or you won't have room to shake the dressings when you are ready to eat. Seal the lid on & store in the fridge. When ready (with the lid on) shake the jar to mix everything.

Roast chicken Salad-in-a-jar

This fills one 32 oz. Mason jar. Make sure to wash & dry your veggies before using.

3 Tbsp. balsamic Vinaigrette

½ cup button mushrooms, sliced

¼ cup cherry tomatoes

½ of a red onion, minced

½ cup cooked, cold roasted chicken, diced

¼ cup organic romaine lettuce

Place the dressing in the bottom of the jar. Next add the mushrooms, add the tomatoes, add the onions, add the roast chicken and then add the chopped romaine. To make it easier on me, I buy a whole, hot roasted chicken from the deli at my local grocery store. Try not to pack it in too tight, or you won't have room to shake the dressings when you are ready to eat. Seal the lid on & store in the fridge. When ready (with the lid on) shake the jar to mix everything.

Balsamic Vinaigrette

3 tablespoons balsamic vinegar

1 tablespoon Dijon mustard

1 garlic clove, minced

1/2 cup olive oil

Salt and freshly ground pepper

In a small bowl, combine the vinegar, mustard, and garlic. Add the oil in a slow steady stream, whisking constantly. Season with salt and pepper to taste.

Layered Taco Salad-in-a-jar

This fills one 32 oz. Mason jar. Make sure to wash & dry your veggies before using.

¼ cup cucumber, diced

1 roma tomato, diced

½ cup black beans, rinsed and drained

¼ cup corn

¼ red bell pepper, diced

¼ cup avocado, diced

1 cup of romaine lettuce, chopped

2 tablespoon of goat cheese

Cilantro-lime dressing

1 tablespoon apple cider vinegar

Juice from 1 lime

½ cup fresh cilantro

¼ cup nonfat Greek yogurt (I have a recipe for nondairy yogurt in the back) 1 teaspoon raw honey

Blend the salad dressing until smooth and pour it in the bottom of your mason jar. Next layer you salad from heaviest to lightest. Add your cucumbers, then your tomatoes, next your black beans and your corn. On top of that place your red bell pepper, next your avocado. Lastly place your lettuce and then the cheese on top of that. Try not to pack it in too tight, or you won't have room to shake the dressings when you are ready to eat. Seal the lid on & store in the fridge. When ready (with the lid on) shake the jar to mix everything.

Grilled Chicken, Beet, Apple Salad-in –a-jar

This fills one 32 oz. Mason jar. Make sure to wash & dry your veggies before using.

1 beets, scrubbed, peeled and diced into small bite size pieces

1 teaspoon olive oil

Salt and pepper to taste

¼ cup roasted chicken breast, diced

1/2 apple, washed and diced

2 cups organic romaine lettuce

1 ounce goat cheese

¼ cup raw pumpkin seeds

Strawberry Vinaigrette

1/4 cup fresh strawberries

1/2 tablespoon olive oil

1/2 tablespoon balsamic vinegar

Pinch of salt

Pinch of ground black pepper

1/4 teaspoon raw honey

Blend the salad dressing until smooth and pour it in the bottom of your mason jar. Next layer you salad from heaviest to lightest. Add your beets, then your chicken and your diced apples. Lastly place your lettuce, next the goat cheese, then your raw pumpkin seeds. Try not to pack it in too tight, or you won't have room to shake the dressings when you are ready to eat. Seal the lid on & store in the fridge. When ready (with the lid on) shake the jar to mix everything.

Smoked Salmon Salad-a-Jar

This fills one 32 oz. Mason jar. Make sure to wash & dry your veggies before using.

¼ cup smoked salmon, diced

¼ cup cucumbers, diced

2 carrots shredded

¼ cup red onion, diced

2 cups organic romaine lettuce

Lemony vinaigrette

3 tablespoons olive oil

1 tablespoon white balsamic vinegar

1/2 Meyer lemon, zested and juiced

In a small bowl, whisk together olive oil, vinegar, lemon juice, and of lemon juice with the zest. Pour in the bottom of your mason jar.

Next add the cucumbers, carrots, red onion, salmon and lettuce. Try not to pack it in too tight, or you won't have room to shake the dressings when you are ready to eat. Seal the lid on & store in the fridge. When ready (with the lid on) shake the jar to mix everything.

Spring Artichoke Salad

1/4 pound red potatoes, quartered

1/2 pound green beans, cut into 2-inch pieces

2- 6 oz. jars marinated artichoke quarters (keep 2 Tablespoons of the marinade)

3 Tablespoons olive oil

2 Tablespoons fresh lemon juice

1 teaspoon Dijon mustard

2 Tablespoons parsley, chopped

2 teaspoons dried oregano

2 teaspoons orange zest

1 cup cherry tomatoes, halved

Salt, to taste

Pepper, to taste

Blanch your green beans in a boiling water green beans until crisp and tender, about 1 minute. Remove the beans from the hot water with a slotted spoon and place in a bowl of cold water. After you've removed the beans add your diced red potatoes to the same water and allow them to cook until they are tender. Next, remove the beans from the cold water after a minute this stops the cooking process and pat the beans dry to remove excess water. Once the potatoes have cooked for about 8 minutes, remove them from the water and drain. Drain the liquid out of the artichoke hearts, reserving 2 Tablespoons of the marinade. In a bowl, add the reserved 2 Tablespoons of artichoke marinade, plus the olive oil, lemon juice, Dijon mustard, parsley and oregano. Whisk together until combined. Next add the potatoes, green beans, artichoke hearts and cherry tomatoes to the bowl of dressing and toss to combine well. Season with your Himalayan sea salt or Celtic sea salt and pepper to taste. Serve chilled or at room temperature.

Quinoa Chickpea and Avocado Salad

1 cup quartered grape tomatoes

15-ounce can garbanzo beans, rinsed and drained

1 cup cooked quinoa

2 tablespoon red onion, minced

2 tablespoon cilantro, minced

1 1/2 limes, juiced

Himalayan sea salt or Celtic sea salt

1 cup diced cucumber

4 oz. diced avocado (1 medium Hass)

Combine all the ingredients except for avocado and cucumber. Next season with salt and pepper to taste. Keep refrigerated until ready to serve. Just Before serving, add cucumber and avocado.

Smoked Turkey Salad-in-a-Jar

This fills one 32 oz. Mason jar. Make sure to wash & dry your veggies before using.

3 tablespoons of raspberry balsamic vinaigrette

¼ cup smoked turkey, diced

¼ cup cucumbers, diced

¼ cup cherry tomatoes, diced

2 boiled eggs, diced

5 tbsp. Walnuts, raw

2 cups organic romaine lettuce

Raspberry Vinaigrette Dressing

1 cup of fresh raspberries

¼ cup olive oil

2/3 cup balsamic vinegar

1 tablespoon of honey

Blend everything until smooth.

Pour 3 tablespoons of the vinaigrette in the bottom of your mason jar. Next add your cucumbers, cherry tomatoes, turkey, romaine lettuce, boiled eggs and walnuts. Try not to pack it in too tight, or you won't have room to shake the dressings when you are ready to eat. Seal the lid on & store in the fridge. When ready (with the lid on) shake the jar to mix everything

Cajun Shrimp salad-in-a-jar

¼ cup sautéed bell peppers, diced

¼ cup sautéed onions, diced

¼ cup Cajun shrimp, cooked

¼ cup freshly smashed guacamole

½ cup Boston Bibb lettuce

Sautee your bell peppers and onions in extra virgin olive oil. Set aside. Next sauté your shrimp in dash of paprika, garlic granules, chili powder, cayenne, and Himalayan sea salt. Cook until completely pink. You want to buy shrimp that is already deveined and the tails are cut off.

Sweet Potato Soup

2lbs of sweet potatoes, chopped

1 onion, diced

1 carrot, diced

1 tsp of minced garlic

3 cups of chicken stock

½ cup coconut milk

Place everything in a slow cooker except for the coconut milk. Cook on low for 6 or high for 4. Puree smooth then add the coconut milk and cook an additional 30 minutes.

Slow Cooker Quinoa, Chicken and Butternut Squash Soup

1 medium butternut squash, peeled and cubed

14 oz. can coconut milk, full fat

2 cups water

2 tbsp. raw honey or maple syrup

1 tbsp. red curry paste

1 inch ginger, peeled & grated

1 garlic clove, crushed

1 1/2 tsp salt

1.5 lbs. chicken breast

2 cups quinoa, cooked

2 large red bell peppers, thinly sliced

1/4 cup cilantro, chopped

1/2 lime, juice of

In a large slow cooker, add squash, coconut milk, water, honey, curry paste, ginger, garlic, salt, lime leaves and chicken. Cover and cook on Low for 8 hours or on High for 4 hours. Remove chicken and shred using two forks. Using immersion blender, blend soup until smooth. Add chicken, quinoa, bell peppers, cilantro and lime juice. Stir and enjoy!

"Creamy" Chicken Tomato Soup Slow Cooker

4 frozen skinless boneless chicken breast

Garlic salt to taste

2 tablespoons Italian Seasoning

1 tablespoon dried basil

1 clove garlic

1 14 oz. can of coconut milk (full fat)

1 14 oz. can diced tomatoes and juice

1 cup of chicken broth

Sea Salt and pepper to taste

Put all the above ingredients into the crock-pot, cook for 9 hours on low. After 9 hours take two forks and shred the chicken, set the crock-pot on warm till ready to serve. For a creamier soup, before adding back the shredded chicken. Blend some of the soup and put it back in the slow cooker. You can this in batches in a regular blend but remember it's hot or use an immersion hand held blender.

Main dishes

Spaghetti Squash & Turkey Meatballs

1 3-pound spaghetti squash

2 tablespoons water

2 tablespoons extra-virgin olive oil, divided

1/2 cup chopped fresh parsley, divided

1 1/4 teaspoons Italian seasoning, divided

1/2 teaspoon onion powder

1/2 teaspoon salt, divided

1/2 teaspoon freshly ground pepper

1 pound 93%-lean ground turkey

4 large cloves garlic, minced

1 28-ounce can no-salt-added crushed tomatoes

1/4-1/2 teaspoon crushed red pepper

Halve squash lengthwise and scoop out the seeds. Place face down in a microwave-safe dish; add ¼ cup water. Microwave, uncovered, on High until the flesh can be easily scraped with a fork, 10 to 15 minutes.

Heat 1 tablespoon oil in a large skillet over medium-high heat. Scrape the squash flesh into the skillet and cook, stirring occasionally, until the moisture is evaporated and the squash is beginning to brown, 5 to 10 minutes. Stir in 1/4 cup parsley. Remove from heat, cover and let stand.

Meanwhile, combine the remaining 1/4 cup parsley, 1/2 teaspoon Italian seasoning, onion powder, 1/4 teaspoon salt and pepper in a medium bowl. Add turkey; gently mix to combine (do not overmix). Using about 2 tablespoons each, form into 12 meatballs.

Heat the remaining 1 tablespoon oil in a large nonstick skillet over medium-high heat. Add the meatballs, reduce heat to medium and cook, turning occasionally, until browned all over, 4 to 6 minutes. Push the meatballs to the side of the pan, add garlic and cook, stirring, for 1 minute. Add tomatoes, crushed red pepper to taste, the remaining 3/4 teaspoon Italian seasoning and 1/4 teaspoon salt; stir to coat the meatballs. Bring to a simmer, cover and cook, stirring occasionally, until the meatballs are cooked through, 10 to 12 minutes more.

Serve the sauce and meatballs over the squash.

Garlic Shrimp with Cilantro Spaghetti Squash

1 2 1/2- to 3-pound spaghetti squash, halved lengthwise and seeded

2 tablespoons extra-virgin olive oil

1 tablespoon minced garlic

1 teaspoon ground coriander

1 teaspoon ground cumin

1/2 teaspoon salt, divided

1/4 teaspoon cayenne pepper

1/3 cup dry white wine

1 pound peeled and deveined raw shrimp (16-20 per pound), tails left on if desired

1 tablespoon lemon juice

1/4 cup chopped fresh cilantro

2 tablespoons non-dairy butter, melted

1/4 teaspoon ground pepper

Lemon wedges for serving

Halve squash lengthwise and scoop out the seeds. Place face down in a microwave-safe dish; add ¼ cup water. Microwave, uncovered, on High until the flesh can be easily scraped with a fork, 10 to 15 minutes. Next heat oil in a large skillet over medium-high heat. Add garlic, coriander, cumin, 1/4 teaspoon salt and cayenne; cook, stirring, for 30 seconds. Add wine and bring to a simmer. Add shrimp and cook, stirring, until the shrimp are pink and just cooked through, 3 to 4 minutes. Remove from heat and stir in lemon juice.

Use a fork to scrape the squash from the shells into a medium bowl. Add cilantro, butter, pepper and the remaining 1/4 teaspoon salt; stir to combine. Serve the shrimp over the spaghetti squash with a lemon wedge on the side.

Oven-Fried Salmon Cakes over a bed of Quinoa Pilaf

1 (14.75 ounce) can wild-caught pink or red salmon

1 cup cooked (or canned) sweet potato, mashed

2 large eggs, beaten

1/2 cup almond flour

1/2 cup fresh parsley leaves, minced (about 2 tablespoons)

2 scallions, white and green, very thinly sliced

1 tablespoon Old Bay Seasoning

1 teaspoon salt

1 teaspoon hot sauce

1/2 teaspoon paprika

1/4 teaspoon ground black pepper

Zest from 1 lemon

2 tablespoons non-dairy butter, melted

Preheat the oven to 425F and cover a large baking sheet with parchment paper. Drain the liquid from the salmon and using your fingers, crumble the fish into a large mixing bowl, removing the bones and flaking the fish. Add the sweet potato, eggs, almond flour, parsley, scallions, Old Bay Seasoning, salt, hot pepper sauce, paprika, black pepper, and lemon zest. Mix well and refrigerate for 10 minutes.

Brush the parchment paper with some of the melted non-dairy butter, then use a 1/3 measuring cup to scoop the cakes and drop them onto the parchment. The patties should be about 2 1/2 inches wide and about 1 inch thick. Brush the tops of the cakes with the nondairy butter, then bake for 20 minutes. Carefully flip each patty with a spatula and return to the oven. Bake an additional 10 minutes until golden brown and crisp. Serve with a squeeze of lemon juice and your sauce of choice.

Baked chicken and sweet potato casserole

1lb of chicken, cubed and diced

2 teaspoon of mustard

3tablepoons of evvo

2 medium sweet potatoes, peeled and diced

Salt & pepper to season

Preheat oven to 425. Diced your chicken into cubes and mix the diced chicken in a bowl with mustard and evoo. Sautee your diced chicken in a pan until it is no longer pink on the outside. Place your precooked chicken in a baking dish. Mix your diced sweet potatoes with your chicken. Season with salt n pepper and cook for 25 minutes until sweet potatoes are tender & chicken is cooked through.

Artichoke Rosemary Chicken

4 lb boneless, skinless chicken breast (trimmed of any extra tendons or fat) and cut into thirds

4 fresh artichoke hearts (halved) or 2 cups of canned artichoke hearts

1 medium red onion, sliced

1 lb. baby portabella mushrooms, halved or quartered

4 Tbsp. horseradish mustard or brown mustard

6-8 cloves fresh garlic, minced

1/4 cup extra virgin olive oil

1/2 cup balsamic vinegar

1/2 cup white wine

1 teaspoon dried basil

1/2 teaspoon dried thyme

1 teaspoon dried rosemary

Himalayan sea salt and black pepper to taste

Place your cut up chicken in a large glass casserole baking pan. Evenly place the artichoke hearts, onions, and mushrooms. Sprinkle to taste with pepper and salt.

In a small bowl mix together the mustard, garlic, olive oil, balsamic vinegar, white wine, basil, thyme, and rosemary. Pour the liquid over the chicken/artichoke/onions. Bake at 350 degrees for 75 minutes. Serve with brown rice or rosemary sweet potatoes.

One pot Skillet chili mac n cheese

1 tablespoon olive oil

2 cloves garlic, minced

1 onion diced

1 red bell pepper, diced

1 lb. of grass fed beef

4 cups of low sodium chicken broth

1 (14.5) toasted diced tomatoes

1 can of white kidney beans, rinsed well

1 can of red kidney beans, rinsed well

3 teaspoons of chili powder

10 ounces of uncooked elbow brown rice pasta

¾ cup of goats cheese

Place your EVOO in a large skillet or Dutch oven over medium heat. Add garlic, onion and ground beef, and cook until browned, about 3-5 minutes, making sure to crumble the beef as it cooks; drain excess fat. Next pour in chicken broth, tomatoes, beans, chili powder and cumin; season with salt n pepper. Bring to a simmer & stir in pasta. Reduce heat and cover allow to simmer for 15 minutes until pasta is tender.

One Pan Ranch Pork Chops and Veggies

4 (8-ounce) pork chops, bone-in, 3/4-inch to 1-inch thick

16 ounces baby red potatoes, halved

16 ounces green beans, trimmed

2 tablespoons olive oil

1 (1-ounce) package Ranch Seasoning and Salad Dressing Mix

3 cloves garlic, minced

Himalayan sea salt and freshly ground black pepper, to taste

2 tablespoons chopped fresh parsley leaves

Preheat oven to 400 degrees F. Lightly oil a baking pan.

Place pork chops, potatoes and green beans in a single layer onto the prepared baking pan. Drizzle with olive oil and sprinkle with Ranch Seasoning and garlic; season with salt and pepper, to taste.

Place into oven and roast until the pork is completely cooked through, reaching an internal temperature of 140 degrees F, about 20-22 minutes. Next turn on the broiler and broil for 2-3 minutes, or until caramelized and slightly charred.

Garlic Zucchini Noodles w/ meat balls

2 zucchinis, cleaned

1 tablespoon EVOO

¼ teaspoon garlic powder

¼ teaspoon garlic salt

1 pound lean ground chicken, turkey or beef

4 large cloves garlic, minced

1 28-ounce can no-salt-added crushed tomatoes

1/4-1/2 teaspoon crushed red pepper

Pepper to taste

Spiralize your zucchini.

Meanwhile, combine the remaining 1/4 cup parsley, 1/2 teaspoon Italian seasoning, onion powder, 1/4 teaspoon salt and pepper in a medium bowl. Add ground chicken. ; Gently mix to combine (do not overmix). Using about 2 tablespoons each, form into 12 meatballs.

Heat the remaining 1 tablespoon oil in a large nonstick skillet over medium-high heat. Add the meatballs, reduce heat to medium and cook, turning occasionally, until browned all over, 4 to 6 minutes. Push the meatballs to the side of the pan, add garlic and cook, stirring, for 1 minute. Add tomatoes, crushed red pepper to taste, the remaining 3/4 teaspoon Italian seasoning and 1/4 teaspoon salt; stir to coat the meatballs. Bring to a simmer, cover and cook, stirring occasionally, until the meatballs are cooked through, 10 to 12 minutes more.

In another skillet on the stove over medium heat.

Once pan is hot, add EVOO and zoodles. Let sauté for about a minute, then add in the seasonings. Cook additional 2-3 minutes. Zoodles should be soft, but still have a slight stiffness. Next incorporate the zoodles and the meatball/sauce mixture and gentle mix.

Oven Baked Fajita

1 pound boneless, skinless chicken breasts, cut into strips

2 Tbsp. coconut oil, melted

2 tsp chili powder

1 1/2 tsp cumin

1/2 tsp garlic powder

1/2 tsp dried oregano

1/4 tsp seasoned salt

1 (15 oz) can diced tomatoes with green chilies

1 medium onion, sliced

1/2 red bell pepper, cut into strips

1/2 green bell pepper, cut into strips

Place chicken strips in a greased 13×9 baking dish. Preheat your oven to 400 degrees.

In a bowl mix the oil, chili powder, cumin, garlic powder, dried oregano, and salt.

Mix the seasoning over the chicken and stir to coat.

Next add the tomatoes, peppers, and onions to the dish and stir to combine.

Bake uncovered for 20-25 minutes or until chicken is cooked through and the vegetables are tender. You can eat this in a large lettuce leaf.

Snacks

Coconut Flour Cupcakes

½ cup melted coconut oil

⅔ Cup coconut sugar

½ teaspoon Himalayan salt

2 teaspoons vanilla extract

6 large eggs

2 Tablespoons water

½ cup coconut flour

1 teaspoon baking powder

Preheat your oven to 350º. Whisk oil sugar, salt, vanilla, eggs, and water. Next add in the coconut flour and baking powder. Add your egg mixture in with the flour mixture and make sure its combined well. Place a dozen paper cupcake in your muffin pan. Fill each cup ¾ full. Bake your cupcakes on the center rack of the oven for 18-20 minutes, until a toothpick inserted into the center of a cupcake comes out clean. After you remove the cupcakes from oven allow them to cool for 5 minutes. Make sure you allow them to cool completely before you add your icing.

Banana-Coconut Raw Vegan Ice Cream

6 bananas, frozen and cut into pieces

½ cup shredded coconut

¼ teaspoon 100% Pure Vanilla Powder

Place your bananas in a high speed blender. I have a Vitamix but a food processor will work too. Blend until they're smooth and creamy. Don't blend for too long or the ice cream will begin to melt. Next add the shredded coconut and vanilla and blend for 30 seconds or until the coconut and vanilla are thoroughly mixed into the ice cream. Serve in bowls and you can add melted chocolate or other toppings on top!

Dark Chocolate coconut apricot bites

5 dried Apricots

1/2 ounce dark chocolate

Sprinkle some coarse Celtic sea salt and shredded coconut

Lay a piece of parchment paper on a plate. Heat dark chocolate in a small bowl in the microwave at 20 second intervals. Stir often and heat until JUST melted (chocolate burns easily in the microwave). Dip 1/2 apricot in the chocolate, put on plate, and dust with salt. Refrigerate for 1/2 hour and serve.

No-bake oatmeal bites

 1 cup dry quick oats

 2/3 cup coconut flakes

 1/2 cup almond butter

  1/2 cup dark chocolate chips

1/3 cup raw honey

1 tsp vanilla

Directions: Mix all ingredients, form into 1 inch balls. Place balls in refrigerator and snack away.

Fried Chickpeas

2 teaspoons smoked paprika

1 teaspoon cayenne pepper

6 tablespoons extra-virgin olive oil

2 15-oz. cans chickpeas, rinsed, drained, patted very dry

Kosher salt

2 teaspoons finely grated lime zest

Combine paprika and cayenne in a small bowl and set aside.

Heat oil in a cast iron skillet over medium-high heat. Working in 2 batches, add chickpeas to skillet and sauté, stirring frequently, until golden and crispy, 15–20 minutes. Using a slotted spoon, transfer chickpeas to paper towels to get excess oil off. Transfer to a bowl. Sprinkle paprika mixture over; toss to coat. Season to taste with salt. Toss with lime zest and serve. You can eat this over a bowl of brown rice or quinoa.

Spicy pumpkin seeds

Dash of Himalayan sea salt

1 teaspoon of coconut oil

¼ teaspoon of smoked paprika

¼ teaspoon of garlic powder

1/8 teaspoon of chili powder

1 cup of raw pumpkin seeds

Melt coconut oil. Mix everything with the seeds in a bowl. Lay seeds on a baking dish. Roast for 20 minutes tossing after 10. Make sure they don't become overly brown. That means the inside of the seed is burning.

Salad Dressings

Many over-the-counter condiments, sauces and salad dressings are filled with Trans fats, sugar, preservatives, and artificial ingredients and flavors. You will be amazed if you started to read labels. You would see words like calcium disodium EDTA, canola oil (and/or soybean oil), caramel color, cellulose gum, cornstarch (or modified cornstarch), disodium guanylate, disodium inosinate, gum arabic, MSG (monosodium glutamate), polysorbate 60, potassium sorbate, sodium and calcium caseinates. Making your own condiments, sauces and salad dressings is easy. All it takes is a little extra time. Do you want your condiments, sauces or salad dressing to come from a lab or your kitchen? All the recipes can be prepared ahead and refrigerated in a mason jar with a tightly sealed lid up to 1 week. You can find more of these mouthwatering recipes in my book **A Survivors Guide to kicking Hypothyroidism Booty.**

Red Wine Vinaigrette

2 tablespoons red wine vinegar

1 teaspoon Dijon mustard (optional)

1 small garlic clove, minced (optional)

1/3 cup extra-virgin olive oil

Coarse salt and ground pepper

Pour all the ingredients in a mason jar with a lid and give a good shake to combine. You can season with Himalayan sea salt and freshly ground black pepper. Store in refrigerator

Honey-Balsamic Vinaigrette

2 tablespoons balsamic vinegar

1 tablespoon raw honey

1 teaspoon Dijon mustard

1/4 cup extra-virgin olive oil

1 garlic glove, minced

Freshly ground black pepper and Himalayan Sea salt to taste. Pour all the ingredients in a mason jar with a lid and give a good shake to combine. You can season with Himalayan sea salt and freshly ground black pepper. Store in refrigerator.

Basic Vinaigrette

1 cup olive oil

1/4 cup organic apple cider vinegar

1 teaspoon garlic powder

1 teaspoon onion powder

1 teaspoon Celtic sea salt

1/2 teaspoon black pepper

Pour all the ingredients in a mason jar with a lid and give a good shake to combine. You can season with Himalayan sea salt and freshly ground black pepper. Store in refrigerator.

Cucumber–Coconut Milk Ranch Dressing

1 can full-fat coconut milk or coconut cream,

Refrigerated overnight

1 medium cucumber, peeled, halved lengthwise, seeded, and

Grated on the large holes of a box grater

2 tablespoons minced shallots

1 garlic clove, minced

2 tablespoons organic apple cider vinegar

3 tablespoons chopped fresh chives

1 1/2 tablespoons chopped fresh parsley

1 1/2 tablespoons chopped fresh basil

1 tablespoon chopped fresh dill

Pinch of cayenne pepper

Place a can of full-fat coconut milk in the fridge overnight this will help the cull-fat of the coconut milk go to the store and be easy to scoop out. After you've done this scoop cream off the top of the can and add it to a large mason jar. Save 4 tablespoons of the coconut water in the can and add it to the hard coconut cream and mix together until smooth. Don't discard the other coconut water. If the mixture is thick you always add more coconut to thin it out. Add the remaining ingredients to your mason jar. Close lid tightly, shake until combined and refrigerate dressing for at least 30 minutes to let the flavors combine together. Keep in the refrigerator after you use it to remain fresh.

What has this book taught me?

1. You need to keep a food and stress journal.
2. Take your thyroid medication with warm lemon water
3. Limit your caffeine
4. Substitute coffee for Matcha tea or a good herbal tea
5. Eat a wholesome, hearty breakfast no later than 2 hours of waking up
6. Read labels
7. Why you need to limit certain vegetables
8. Avoid soy, gluten products, processed foods, artificial additives, chemical laden products
9. How to start making your own cleaning products-very easy
10. Why you should start taking probiotics, digestive enzymes and the correct vitamins
11. Get some sunlight!
12. Why you should have a healthy gut and how to accomplish that
13. Why you should wait 4 hours before taking supplements after your thyroid medication
14. How to start coping with stress
15. How to not get bored with exercise
16. Foods that you need to eat
17. Easy to make recipes
18. Change your cookware from Teflon pans to stainless steel, ceramic or cast iron.
19. Be grateful, be happy, be yourself, you can do this, I believe in you.

Tell me what you eat, and I will tell you what you are.

— Anthelme Brillat-Savarin (1755–1826)

The Physiology of Taste

Hot Mess to Great Success

Audrey's Hypothyroidism's Journey

After being diagnosed with hypothyroidism over 10 years ago. I knew, there was something more than just being labeled with a medical condition. There wasn't a lot of information on how to heal myself from the inside out. Google, Amazon or Facebook wasn't invented yet. I decided to give myself permission, on this road of life that I've traveling so blindly. I soon realize that I am responsibility for my own life. I can't sit around waiting for someone to fix me. I wasn't wasting my time because I have the power to take responsibility to move my life forward. I figured out that part of my purpose and part of my journey was to be able to look back on my path of life and to accept what I've learned. I realized that there were other people who were also on this same journey as me. Who although they might not be exactly where I am in my journey but people who might not know exactly what I know and they do want to know. They need to know. We all have a voice. We are our own best advocate in life. We must never stop finding out truths, walking our destiny and making a positive difference in this world. Who would have thought that a girl whose favorite subjects in school was lunch and boys would suddenly be a research for the truth, a writer for the unspoken, a health journalist to the unknown and published author to all.

I am unique. I own my awesomeness. I deserve to be happy and successful. You do too. The late great Bernie Mac was not only a wonderful actor, comedian but also a brilliant visionary who spoke the truth. Oprah asked him: "What did you think what your goal was?" He replies: "I want to be the best within myself. I am not in competition with anybody. If you focus on being the best within yourself all that stuff will come. Money shouldn't be you motivation. If you do well then money will come. I am not a black comedian. I am a comedian. I want to make everyone laugh." This is how I feel. I want to be the best that I can be. I am focused on being the best at empowering people to embrace who they are, to add voice to their life, to inspire them and to connect with all those who are struggling with hypothyroidism.

I love this statement by Mark Macdonald, Co-Ceo and Co-founder of Appster.

I believe that you should make a habit of believing in the things that people think are impossible. Learn to question everything. Experts will always try to convince you that what you want to do is impossible and simply won't work. However, every successful endeavor starts with one stubborn person who refuses to operate by the same rules and type of thinking that everyone else does.

Be that person.

About the Author

A. L. Childers is an inspiring author, blogger and health journalist. She is the creator and founder of the website: Thehypothyroidismchick.com. Where you can find great tips on everyday living with hypothyroidism. She has tried every diet out there - twice. After pledging to give up yo-yo dieting and fad diets, she solemnly swore never to look back. She believes that everyone deserves the chance to live a healthy lifestyle. She has done the research and is giving you the blueprint to achieve your goals.

A.L. Enjoys dancing, a nice bottle of blended red wine and spending quality time with close friends and family. She has also written **Reset Your Thyroid: A 21 day reboot program, The Survivors guide to Kicking hypothyroidisms booty and The Survivors Cookbook Guide to Kicking Hypothyroidisms Booty: The Slow Cooker Way.** You can also find her on Instagram and twitter @ thyroidismchick and her face book page Healing Hypothyroidism.

Resources:

The American Institute for Cancer Research. The New American Plate: A timely approach to eating for healthy life and healthy weight.

Fung, T. T. et al. Association between dietary patterns and plasma biomarkers of obesity and cardiovascular disease risk. American Journal of Clinical Nutrition, January 2001. 73:61–67.

Centers for Disease Control. Overweight. April 2006. http://www.cdc.gov/nchs/fastats/overwt.htm

Alliance for a Healthier Generation. Alliance for a Healthier Generation Clinton Foundation and American Heart Association and Industry Leaders Set Healthy School Beverage Guidelines for US Schools. May 2006.

US Department of Agriculture. How much food from the meat and bans group is needed daily? http://www.mypyramid.gov/pyramid/meat_amount.aspx

Ogden, CL et al. High Body Mass Index for Age Among US Children and Adolescents, 2003-2006. Journal of the American Medical Association. 299(20):2401-2405. May 2008. http://jama.amaassn.org/cgi/content/short/299/20/2401

Higdon J, Delage B, Williams D, et al: Cruciferous vegetables and human cancer risk: epidemiologic evidence and mechanistic basis. Pharmacol Res 2007;55:224–236.

Wu QJ, Yang Y, Vogtmann E, et al: Cruciferous vegetables intake and the risk of colorectal cancer: a meta-analysis of observational studies. Ann Oncol 2012.

Liu X, Lv K: Cruciferous vegetables intake is inversely associated with risk of breast cancer: A meta-analysis. Breast 2012.

Liu B, Mao Q, Lin Y, et al: The association of cruciferous vegetables intake and risk of bladder cancer: a meta-analysis. World JUrol 2012.

Liu B, Mao Q, Cao M, et al: Cruciferous vegetables intake and risk of prostate cancer: a meta-analysis. Int J Urol 2012;19:134–141.

Lam TK, Gallicchio L, Lindsley K, et al: Cruciferous vegetable consumption and lung cancer risk: a systematic review. Cancer Epidemiol Biomarkers Prev 2009;18:184–195.

Bosetti C, Negri E, Kolonel L, et al: A pooled analysis of case-control studies of thyroid cancer. VII. Cruciferous and other vegetables (International). Cancer Causes Control 2002;13:765–775.

Dal Maso L, Bosetti C, La Vecchia C, et al: Risk factors for thyroid cancer: an epidemiological review focused on nutritional factors. Cancer Causes Control 2009;20:75–86.

Phytochemicals and Other Dietary Factors 2nd edition: Thieme; 2013

Krajcovicova-Kudlackova M, Buckova K, Klimes I, et al: Iodine deficiency in vegetarians and vegans. Ann Nutr Metab 2003; 47:183–185.

Leung AM, Lamar A, He X, et al: Iodine status and thyroid function of Boston-area vegetarians and vegans. J Clin Endocrinol Metab 2011;96:E1303–1307.

Office of Dietary Supplements, National Institutes of Health. Dietary Supplement Fact Sheet: Iodine.

Tonstad S, Nathan E, Oda K, et al: Vegan diets and hypothyroidism. Nutrients 2013;5:4642–4652.

McMillan M, Spinks EA, Fenwick GR: Preliminary observations on the effect of dietary brussels sprouts on thyroid function. Hum

Toxicol 1986;5:15–19.

Chu M, Seltzer TF: Myxedema coma induced by ingestion of raw bok choy. N Engl J Med 2010;362:1945–1946.

Zhang X, Shu XO, Xiang YB, et al: Cruciferous vegetable consumption is associated with a reduced risk of total and cardiovascular disease mortality. Am J Clin Nutr 2011;94:240–246.

Fenwick GR, Heaney RK, Mullin WJ. Glucosinolates and their breakdown products in food and food plants. Crit Rev Food Sci Nutr. 1983;18(2):123–201

Chu M, Seltzer TF. Myxedema coma induced by ingestion of raw bok choy. N Engl J Med. 2010;362(20):1945–1946.

http://www.mercola.com/Downloads/bonus/dangers-of-nonstick-cookware/report.aspx

Takahashi Y, Kipnis DM, Daughaday WH Growth hormone secretion during sleep. J Clin Invest 1968;47:2079–2090.

Weitzman E. D., Fukushima D, Nogeire C, Roffwarg H, Gallagher T. F., Hellman L. Twenty-four hour pattern of the episodic secretion of cortisol in normal subjects. J Clin Endocriol Metab 1971;33:14–22.

Flegal, K. M. et al. Prevalence and Trends in Obesity Among US Adults, 1999–2008 JAMA. 2010;303(3):235–241.

Interviews with Melanie Polk, registered dietitian and director of nutrition education for the American Institute of Cancer Research

Interview with Marion Nestle, Marion Nestle, PhD, MPH, Chair of the Department of Nutrition and Food Studies at New York University

Interview with Barbara Gollman, registered dietitian and spokesperson for the American Dietetic Association

Nestle, M. and M. F. Jacobson. Halting the obesity epidemic: A public health policy approach. Public Health Reports, January/February 2000. 115:12–24.

http://www.nationofchange.org/ultimate-paradox-us-overfed-andmalnourished-nation-1372077901

http://www.aloeit.com/human-engine-our-bodies-health/

http://www.webmd.com/a-to-z-guides/hypothyroidism-topic-overview

http://www.mayoclinic.org/diseases-conditions/hypothyroidism/basics/symptoms/con-20021179

http://www.webmd.com/a-to-z-guides/hypothyroidism-topic-overview

http://hypothyroidmom.com/300-hypothyroidism-symptoms-yesreally/

http://www.womentowomen.com/thyroid-health/hypothyroidsymptoms-2/

http://www.medicinenet.com/hypothyroidism_symptoms/views.htm

http://www.stopthethyroidmadness.com/long-and-pathetic/

Mazokopakis EE, Starakis IK, Papadomanolaki MG, Batistakis AG, Papadakis JA. Changes of bone mineral density in pre-menopausal women with differentiated thyroid cancer receiving L-thyroxine suppressive therapy. Curr Med Res Opin. 2006;22:1369–73. [PubMed]

2. Mandel SJ, Brent GA, Larsen PR. Levothyroxine therapy in patients with thyroid disease. Ann Intern Med. 1993;119:492–502. [PubMed]

3. Singh N, Singh PN, Hershman JM. Effect of calcium carbonate on the absorption of levothyroxine . JAMA. 2000;283:2822–5. [PubMed]

4. Singh N, Weisler SL, Hershman JM. The acute effect of calcium carbonate on the intestinal absorption of levothyroxine. Thyroid. 2001; 11:967–71. [PubMed]

5. Neafsey PJ. Levothyroxine and calcium interaction: timing is everything. Home Health Nurse. 2004; 22:338–9. [PubMed]

6. Mazokopakis EE. Counseling patients receiving levothyroxine (L-T4) and calcium carbonate. Mil Med. 2006;171:vii,1094. [PubMed]

[No authors listed]. Iodine. Monograph. Altern Med Rev 2010; 15(3):273–278.

Leung AM and Braverman LE. Iodine-induced thyroid dysfunction. Curr Opin Endocrinol Diabetes Obes 2012; 19(5): 414–419.

Brahmbhatt SR et al. Thyroid ultrasound is the best prevalence indicator for assessment of iodine deficiency disorders: a study in rural/tribal schoolchildren from Gujarat (Western India). European Journal of Endocrinology 2000;143:37–46.

Brahmbhatt SR et al. Study of biochemical prevalence indicators for the assessment of iodine deficiency disorders in adults at field conditions in Gujarat (India). Asia Pacific J Clin Nutr 2001; 10(1):51–57.

Kris-Etherton PM, et al. Polyunsaturated fatty acids in the food chain in the United States. Am J Clin Nutr 2000; 71(1):179S-188S.

Carrington J. Using hormones to heal traumatic brain injuries. [Internet]. Available at: http://www.lef.org/magazine/mag2012/jan2012_Using-Hormones-Heal-Traumatic-Brain-Injuries_01.htm.

Kresser C. How too much Omega-6 and not enough Omega-3 is making us sick. [Internet]. Available at: http://chriskresser.com/how-too-much-omega-6-and-not-enough-omega-3-is-making-us-sick.

- Panda S, et al. Withania somnifera and Bauhinia purpurea in the regulation of circulating thyroid hormone concentrations in female mice. Journal Ethnopharmacology 1999; 67(2):233-9.

Panda S, et al. Changes in thyroid hormone concentrations after administration of ashwaganda root extract to adult male mice. Journal of Pharmacology 1998; 50:1065-1068.

Kalani A, et al. Ashwagandha root in the treatment of non-classical adrenal hyperplasia. BMJ Case Reports 2012; 10(1136).

Agrawal P, et al. Randomized placebo-controlled, single blind trial of holy basil leaves in patients with noninsulin-dependent diabetes mellitus. Int J Clin Pharmacol Ther 1996; 34(9):406-9.

Gholap S, et al. Hypoglycaemic effects of some plant extracts are possibly mediated through inhibition in corticosteroid concentration. Pharmazie 2004; 59 (11):876-8.

Khan V, et al. A pharmacological appraisal of medicinal plants with antidiabetic potential. J Pharm Bioallied Sci 2012; 4(1):27-42.

Norman A. From vitamin D to hormone D: fundamentals of the vitamin D endocrine system essential for good health. Am J Clin Nutr August 2008; 88(2):491S-499S

http://www.mayoclinic.org/healthy-lifestyle/fitness/in-depth/exercise/art-20048389?pg=2

http://healingthebody.ca/coconut-sugar-a-low-gi-sugar-rich-in-amino-acids-and-b-vitamins/

http://info.visiblebody.com/endocrine-system-hypothalamus-and-pituitary

http://www.progressivehealth.com/low-levels-t3-t4.htm

http://www.fluoridealert.org/wp-content/uploads/merck-1968.pdf

http://fluoridealert.org/issues/health/thyroid/

Recipes (as in the measured list of ingredients) and very short directions on how to combine those ingredients are not protected under the various forms of copyright law. This is because they fall under the designation of being the steps in a procedure and they're explicitly excluded from copyright. Countries which are signatories to either the Berne convention or the Buenos Aires convention use the same basic standard to determine what is and isn't copyrighted although there are small local variations. However, the exclusion on procedures is not a local variation. What can be copyrighted are the more complex directions that usually accompany the list of ingredients in modern recipes. As long as you rewrite any directions to be in your own words you've followed the law. Cooking something from a recipe recorded by someone else and selling it is legal.

www.ingramcontent.com/pod-product-compliance
Lightning Source LLC
Chambersburg PA
CBHW060355190526
45169CB00002B/603